*"The role of caregiver is one we will all p
it will be different for each of us. Here is
advice, profound understanding of how caregiving changes the caregiver, and spiritual support during end-of-life all in one space. Hearing the authors' personal experiences is inspiring and reassuring that no one is perfect, but all are capable of being a caregiver advocate. This book is a tool we all need in our toolbox; the sooner, the better!"*

~ Janet Carter, LMSW, Aging Life Care Manager

"OMG, this book should be in all primary care offices and available to all children, parents, and any caregiver.

The format of this book is phenomenal; such a great way to introduce different stories/scenarios. Personalized experiences, we can all see ourselves in someone else's story. I have found some wonderful advice to help my own patients who are dealing with an aging parent, spouse or family member. Each and every chapter is a wealth of information. I have particularly enjoyed the RESOURCES chapter; it has more information than I even knew about.

The beauty of this book is that it can also be helpful for anyone who is experiencing personal terminal/chronic illness or helping a loved one through this journey, though the book is intended for dementia patients. I found the chapter on the father whose daughter contracted herpes encephalitis to be quite moving. The chapter on driving is excellent and helpful; each chapter is well-written. This book should have been published years ago, really very insightful and helpful for EVERYONE. Sooner or later, we will all walk down this path.

I want to purchase several copies and will have an "office copy" in the waiting room.

Thank you for having me evaluate this book. It is really a treasure."

Best,

~ Dr Mariali Garcia, MD, FACE

"This book is a fantastic resource of information for learning where to start, how to take care at the end of the caregiving journey, and all that matters in between. As I read each chapter, I could relate to some of the strategies used and many I wish I had known about when my mom first started her dementia journey.

Each chapter helps you realize you are not alone. They give great insight into self-care and how to make time to destress. There are so many bits and pieces of how they incorporated things into making life better. I think everyone should have this book. It would allow anyone a jump-start on becoming a caregiver and tools/resources to use along the way. Thank you, and God Bless."

~ Tami Beckett Presley, Retired, Three-time caregiver

"Wow! You all did a great job with this one. I really enjoyed it and plan on making sure my people get ahold of a copy."

~ John A. Lao, LPN, RAC-CT, VWCN, Owner/Founder

"I smiled, I laughed, I cried, as I read each chapter. I realized I was not alone in the storm that I know is coming. My 84-year-old mother-in-law has all the symptoms that were shared in this book, each chapter addressing each issue that we are beginning to witness. Even the denial that the diagnosis is what it is. My wife is having the most difficult time accepting what is inevitable. Knowing Debbie personally and witnessing her struggles and her successes with those she has helped gives me strength to prepare.

I am looking for ways to assist my family with our coming challenges, and this book does it!

The Caregiver's Advocate *has a tremendous message of hope and viable methods of graceful and loving suggestions. It is a journey we do not have to take alone.*"

~ Sam Guiterrez, Management Recruiter, Texas and New Mexico

"*Caregiving is excruciatingly hard, and often, you have no idea where to turn. Reading* The Caregiver's Advocate *feels like sitting together with a caring group of people who can guide you and show you the way to the help and information you need next. They've lived it, and they are willing to share their hard-earned knowledge with you. Like great parents, they want your journey to be easier than theirs was. If you're a caregiver in need of support and resources, this book answers your most urgent questions - and questions you don't even know you have yet.*"

~ Carol Hillegas, Freelance Copywriter, Liberty Copy, LLC

"The Caregiver's Advocate *was such a delightful book to read. So many different ideas and tools. I love the part about music and dance. I believe in my soul; we all have that ability built into us. Thank you so much for helping others who are struggling with what could be such a lost feeling. These are helpful tools. Thank you from the bottom of my heart.*"

~ Pamela Bonta, Caregiver, Texas Health And Environment Alliance

The Caregiver's Advocate

A Complete Guide to Support and Resources

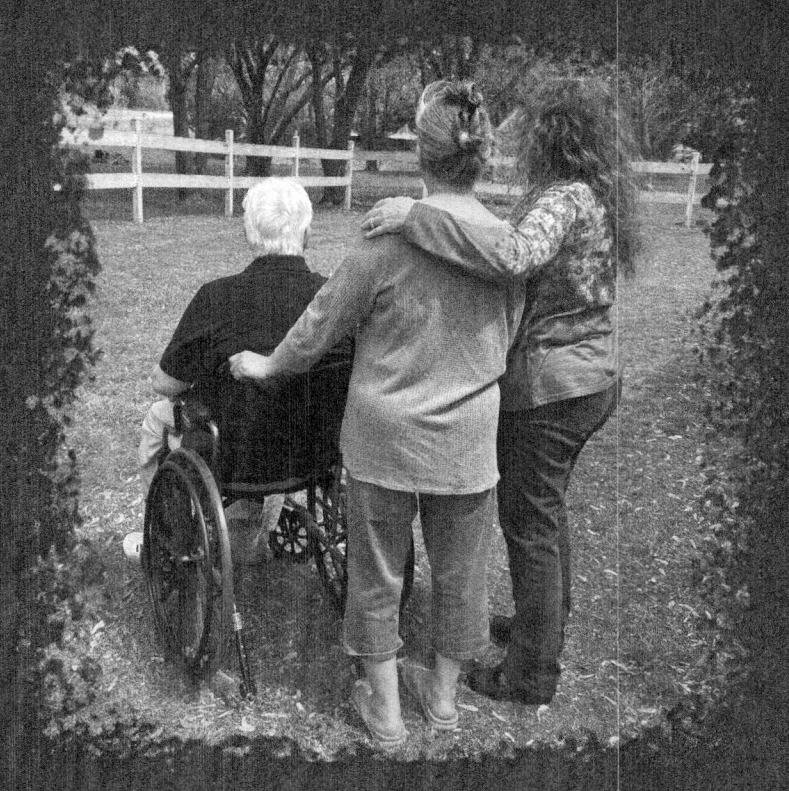

Debbie DeMoss Compton

Featuring: Karen Hulme Alegi, Alexis Baker, Michelle Briggs, Frank Byrum, Ellen Donovan, Daneika D. Farmer, Brenda Freed, Amy Friesen, Diane Marie Gallant, Kathleen Plummer Gordon, R. Scott Holmes, Kim Kasiah, Cheryl M. Kinney, Michael Lewis, Susan J. Ryan, Nicky Sargant, Dr. Carol Sargent, Veronica Scheers, Rev. Dr. Karen Schuder, Rena Yudkowsky

The Caregiver's Advocate

A Complete Guide to Support and Resources

Debbie DeMoss Compton

Featuring: Karen Hulme Alegi, Alexis Baker, Michelle Briggs, Frank Byrum, Ellen Donovan, Daneika D. Farmer, Brenda Freed, Amy Friesen, Diane Marie Gallant, Kathleen Plummer Gordon, R. Scott Holmes, Kim Kasiah, Cheryl M. Kinney, Michael Lewis, Susan J. Ryan, Nicky Sargant, Dr. Carol Sargent, Veronica Scheers, Rev. Dr. Karen Schuder, Rena Yudkowsky

The Caregiver's Advocate
A Complete Guide to Support and Resources

Debbie DeMoss Compton
Copyright © 2024 Debbie DeMoss Compton
Published by Brave Healer Productions
All rights reserved. No part of this book may be used or reproduced by any means, graphic, electronic, or mechanical, including photocopying, recording, taping, or by any information storage retrieval system without the written permission of the publisher, except in the case of brief quotations embodied in critical articles and reviews.

Paperback ISBN: 978-1-961493-31-5

eBook ISBN: 978-1-961493-28-5

Dedication

The Caregiver's Advocate is dedicated to caregivers everywhere. You are the backbone of the health care system, whether you are "just helping out" with Mom and Dad or managing their finances, doctor appointments, and social calendar. You are vital to their longevity.

You may be caring for a special child, your spouse, grandparents, a neighbor, or someone you've just met. Regardless of the specifics, this book is for you.

Each chapter is designed to equip you with valuable information and resources. We've also included our contact information, and we encourage you to let us assist you in making your caregiving journey more manageable.

We are here to help you.

You have a difficult journey with few accolades, so we salute you!

DISCLAIMER

This book offers health and nutritional information and is designed for educational purposes only. You should not rely on this information as a substitute for, nor does it replace professional medical advice, diagnosis, or treatment. If you have any concerns or questions about your health, you should always consult with a physician or other healthcare professional. Do not disregard, avoid, or delay obtaining medical or health-related advice from your healthcare professional because of something you may have read here. The use of any information provided in this book is solely at your own risk.

Developments in medical research may impact the health, fitness, and nutritional advice that appears here. No assurances can be given that the information contained in this book will always include the most relevant findings or developments with respect to the particular material.

Having said all that, know that the experts here have shared their tools, practices, and knowledge with you with a sincere and generous intent to assist you on your health and wellness journey. Please contact them with any questions you may have about the techniques or information they provided. They will be happy to assist you further!

Table of Contents

INTRODUCTION | i

CHAPTER 1

SPARKING JOY AND CONNECTION | 1
SEVEN WAYS TO INFUSE MUSIC INTO DEMENTIA CAREGIVING

By Alexis Baker, MT-BC, CDP

CHAPTER 2

WHEN IT'S TIME FOR THE TALK | 11
TURN AWKWARD CONVERSATIONS
INTO ACTIONABLE ELDERCARE PLANNING

By Amy Friesen, Business and Caregiver Coach

CHAPTER 3

BUILDING YOUR SUPPORT TEAM | 22
THE ART AND FREEDOM OF ASKING FOR AND ACCEPTING HELP

By Cheryl M. Kinney, MSW, LCSW

CHAPTER 4
BE THEIR POWER | 33
LEGAL DOCUMENTS ALL CAREGIVERS NEED
By Karen Hulme Alegi, Attorney

CHAPTER 5
PROMOTE HEALTHY BOUNDARIES TO THRIVE | 41
CREATE BALANCE FOR RESILIENT AND SUSTAINABLE CAREGIVING
By Karen Schuder, EdD, MDiv, MAM

CHAPTER 6
CAREGIVER BURNOUT | 50
WHAT IT IS AND HOW TO AVOID IT
By Debbie DeMoss Compton, CCC, CCA

CHAPTER 7
SAFETY FIRST | 61
WHEN IS IT TIME TO STOP DRIVING?
By Kathleen Plummer Gordon, MSW

CHAPTER 8

THE ART OF FINANCIAL SELF-DEFENSE | 70
STRATEGIES TO PROTECT THE ELDERLY FROM EXPLOITATION
By Michael Lewis, CFA MBA

CHAPTER 9

HANDS-ON CARE | 80
ESSENTIAL TIPS FOR BATHING AND EATING
By Daneika D. Farmer

CHAPTER 10

THE ALZHEIMER'S CONVERSATION | 91
WHY AND HOW TO INCLUDE CHILDREN
By Brenda Freed, MMus

CHAPTER 11

WHY DID I COME TO THE FRIDGE? | 103
FOUR POWERFUL TECHNIQUES TO IMPROVE YOUR MEMORY
By Rena Yudkowsky, MSW, Memory Coach

CHAPTER 12

BE THEIR VOICE | 113
TAKING THE LEAD TO HELP NAVIGATE LATE-LIFE CHALLENGES
By Ellen Donovan, RN, BSN, CDP

CHAPTER 13
A DIFFERENT FEEL | 123
NAVIGATING DEMENTIA SENSORY CHANGES WITH EASE
By Kim Kasiah, PAC Certified Trainer, Coach, and Champion Teacher

CHAPTER 14
FINDING THE GIFT | 132
WHEN CAREGIVING HAS NO END IN SIGHT
By Diane Marie Gallant

CHAPTER 15
STOP THE WORLD; I WANT TO GET OFF! | 144
HOW TO STAY SANE WHILE CARING FOR YOUR LOVED ONE
By R. Scott Holmes

CHAPTER 16
A JOURNEY THROUGH MY MOTHER'S DEMENTIA | 154
HOW TO NAVIGATE THE FOG OF GUARDIANSHIP
By Frank Byrum

CHAPTER 17
ALZHEIMER'S AND REHABILITATION | 163
COULD AN INTEGRATIVE APPROACH BE THE ANSWER?
By Nicky Sargant, Alzheimer's Live-in Carer

CHAPTER 18

LOVE'S RESILIENCE AND HOPE | 175

NAVIGATING MARRIAGE AFTER STROKE AND APHASIA

By Michelle Briggs,
Spouse and Psychiatric Mental Health Nurse Practitioner

CHAPTER 19

FILL YOUR LIFE WITH NEW EXPERIENCES | 181

HOW TO GO ON VACATION WITH YOUR LOVED ONE

By Dr. Carol Sargent

CHAPTER 20

MASSIVE ACCEPTANCE AND RADICAL PRESENCE | 193

THE KEY TO POSITIVELY NAVIGATING
YOUR CAREGIVING JOURNEY

By Susan J. Ryan

CHAPTER 21

HOSPICE AND THE END OF LIFE DOULA | 204

WHEN HOSPICE ISN'T ENOUGH

By Veronica Scheers, RN, CEOLD

CLOSING | 216
WHAT BOAT ARE YOU IN?
By Debbie DeMoss Compton, CCC, CCA

RESOURCES | 222

Introduction

My earliest memory is being on the phone with my mother.

"You have a new baby sister," she told me.

I was so excited! "I'll bring the baby home to meet you in time for your birthday!" My second birthday was in three days.

I grabbed diapers, wipes, and burp cloths with extreme speed and accuracy. Mom counted on me to assist with this tiny, often crying, sweet baby sister, who was so helpless. I was a secondary caregiver at two years old!

A short 15 months later, it happened again!

My mom was a baby-making machine. She had four kids in five years! This time, Mom brought home a baby brother for me to help take care of. I called him my "chubby bubby" because he was a round little guy with an insatiable appetite. By now, I was an expert babysitter, at least in my three-and-a-half-year-old brain.

I adored my younger siblings and enjoyed helping Mom. I had this cute little doll stroller that worked wonderfully for my babies, so one day, I decided to put my chubby little brother in it and take him for a stroll down the hallway.

Things did not go as planned.

His weight was too much for my toy stroller to handle, and the seat quickly split apart, leaving him stuck with his diaper on the ground and feet and arms in the air! I started crying over my beloved stroller lying in ruins.

This was not the plan! We're supposed to have a peaceful stroll down the long hallway. I should not be dealing with a ripped stroller, a screaming baby, and arms and legs flailing wildly. Why is he hitting and kicking me while I'm trying to help him?

While all these emotions were swirling, I knew I had to remedy the situation, so I untangled him from the ripped seat and hoisted him to safety.

Once I freed him, he calmed down and lay there playing with a wheel. I stared at the stroller, trying to decide how best to repair it. I wasn't old enough to use a sewing machine, so I decided on duct tape. I knew it was in the garage, so I grabbed it and quickly taped it around the bars to make a new seat. It worked wonderfully! Dad was less than impressed with the amount I used, but I wanted to be sure he didn't break through again! Problem solved.

My entire life, I learned to use what was available to solve a problem and create a solution.

Just like the duct tape at three and a half years old, I teach people how to react quickly using whatever is at hand to solve a caregiving problem.

Ever feel like you're on your own with no help available? I can help you find help. Have you experienced your loved one punching at you while you're assisting them? I have, and I have solutions.

My name is Debbie Compton, and I'm a three-time caregiver for parents with Alzheimer's, Parkinson's, and Vascular Dementia. I'm a Certified Caregiving Consultant and Certified Caregiver Advocate, Founder of The Purple Vine, keynote speaker, and author of nine books.

My passion is empowering caregivers with tools to reduce stress, block burnout, and laugh again. My website is www.ThePurpleVine.com. On it, you'll find information, resources, and a way to join my tribe.

First, thank you so much for purchasing our book! My co-authors and I all worked hard to bring you valuable, actionable information. Each of us desires to support caregivers, but we approach that differently. Since there isn't a one-size-fits-all solution, we offer a range of things to try. It may work today and not tomorrow, or it may work for a few weeks and then not for a week, or not at all.

We're caregivers of parents, spouses, children, or someone we aren't related to at all. Some of us have also helped care for ailing grandparents. If you are a caregiver, we've all walked the path you're on in one way or another. Most of us learned so much along the journey that we wish we knew initially. Our lives could've been much easier if we knew all the information we're about to share.

We don't want you to struggle like we did. We're motivated to help you. We want you to know we don't judge your bad days or words spoken in haste, perhaps with a less-than-desirable tone. This is a safe space among people who understand. We all make mistakes along the way; you do your best with the information you have. You're not alone.

Each chapter will begin with a personal story relating to the topic. Then, we'll share one or more specific strategies to help you overcome the challenge. These strategies are not theories but actual ways we've managed the situation.

We'll list our contact information at the end of each chapter so you can reach out for more support. Some of us offer counseling or coaching, some have memberships or newsletters you can sign up to receive, and others have products or services. I've collected a range of experts from not only the U.S. but also from Israel, the U.K., and Canada.

Dementia and other diseases recognize no borders. It's a worldwide problem.

Our hope is that by the time you finish reading *The Caregiver's Advocate*, you will have a sustainable plan for caregiving, be encouraged, realize there are millions in the world going through the same thing as you, connect with some or all of the authors, feel a new sense of confidence, and gain valuable resources, strategies, and tools to make your journey less stressful.

Be sure you check out the Resources chapter at the back for companies waiting to help you. They're listed alphabetically by company name, followed by a short blurb and web address.

Sit back, relax, and be prepared to learn new things from people who genuinely care about you.

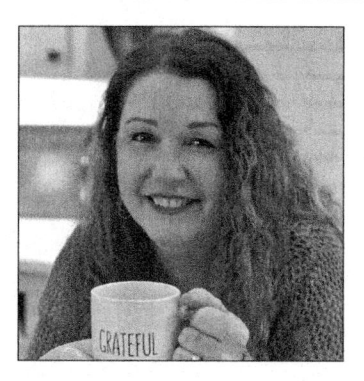

God bless you!

Debbie DeMoss Compton

Deb@ThePurpleVine.com

CHAPTER 1

Sparking Joy and Connection

SEVEN WAYS TO INFUSE MUSIC INTO DEMENTIA CAREGIVING

Alexis Baker, MT-BC, CDP

All I know is that in the midst of the madness of this world, music is my therapy.

- Gordon Lightfoot

MY STORY

"Hey, Mom, let's breathe. Ready? Deep breath in," Charlotte said, reaching for her mom's hand. She inhaled deeply, modeling the action for Beverly. "Deep breath out," she said, making an 'O' shape with her mouth as she exhaled air.

Following her daughter's cues, Beverly inhaled and exhaled deeply, which visibly seemed to help calm the 87-year-old woman.

"Again. Deep breath in," Charlotte spoke gently with a pause and inhale. "Deep breath out." Then she began singing, "Breathing in, breathing out, that's what life is all about," to the melody of Pachelbel's Canon in D, a tune she had learned in their music therapy sessions.

I was honored to meet Charlotte and Beverly through my local chapter of the Alzheimer's Association in Portland, OR. I had the privilege of being their music therapist for about five years before Beverly's passing in late 2022.

When I met Beverly, she was in the later stage of Alzheimer's disease and had mostly lost the ability to speak. She was bed-bound or sat in a wheelchair, and she could do very little for herself. But Beverly was also bright-eyed, pleasant to be with, and had the *best* smile, which I told her often. She would sometimes audibly sing and could mouth song lyrics with me. She could clap, pat her lap, and move to music. She often visibly brightened in response to hearing music and made great eye contact. Best of all, she and her daughter, Charlotte, connected through music. We created beautiful memories by making music together—moments filled with smiles, laughter, and joy.

Initially, I served Beverly at the adult care home where she resided. Charlotte and I would meet there for regular music therapy visits. In June 2019, Charlotte moved Beverly into her home with her, becoming her full-time primary caregiver until the last few months of her life.

Charlotte sought music therapy for Beverly as an enriching activity for her mom. Beverly noticeably benefitted from music therapy, and it also impacted Charlotte. She described to me how music therapy helped her feel empowered by being able to be a part of it. "Having something to provide Mom was a relief on my heart," Charlotte told me. "It was spirit-lifting." She also described it as another tool in her toolbox as a caregiver.

Charlotte is a shining example of incorporating music into the daily care of a loved one with dementia. Outside of our formal music therapy sessions, Charlotte incorporated music at home in many ways. "We had music on quite a bit," she shared. "Benny Goodman, 30's and 40's French jazz, calming soundscapes, even nature sounds." They would dance regularly to help rehabilitate or maintain her mom's range of motion. She used hand-over-hand or hand-under-hand prompting to assist her mom in physical movement.

"Sometimes you just gotta sing it out! Sing what you're thinking or feeling," Charlotte recalled. For example, "You must be frustrated," she said in a sing-song, improvised manner. She would also "sing-explain" what they would do next as a technique to help Beverly transition throughout the day. Charlotte's husband, Michael, plays guitar, and he would play with Beverly. Charlotte's siblings also contributed musically, bringing their various instruments on occasion and singing at family gatherings. Music helped ease the pain of the gradual and eventual loss of their beloved Beverly.

If you would like to see Charlotte and Beverly in action with our program, go here: https://bit.ly/chandbe

THE STRATEGY

One of my ambitions as a music therapist is to encourage, empower, and equip caregivers to incorporate music into the ever-so-important day-to-day of caregiving. Many can be intimidated when something falls outside their comfort zone. In modern American culture, musicality is not always viewed on a spectrum. There are "musicians," and then there are non-musicians. Musical artists are idolized, and we get caught up in this type of thinking: *They're the professionals. I'm not a musician. I'm not talented enough to make music.* On the contrary, **every human is musical in some way**. I stand by this statement.

Did you know music activates every area of the brain? It's true. Scientific researchers have observed that listening to music and engaging in music-based activities can affect all areas of the brain. Music also activates the feel-good centers of the brain, and it can even help create new neural pathways. We're musical beings. Just look at how rhythm is inside each of us: our beating hearts, blood pulsing through our vessels, our rhythmic breathing (in and out, in and out). That's why I believe every human is musical.

Because we're all musical in one way or another, it makes sense to incorporate music into day-to-day caregiving in some way, shape, or form. Music can be a wonderful tool for creating moments of joy and connection. It can help lighten the mood, relieve stress, get you and your loved one moving, increase energy, promote relaxation, and more. Maybe you've never thought of music as a daily activity for you and your loved one, but music is sort of like a vitamin. A little bit every day does wonders to nourish the heart, mind, and soul.

Maybe you're unsure how to utilize music as a meaningful daily activity. My goal with this chapter is to give you practical tips so you walk away ready to try a few new activities. These are easy-to-implement ideas and mainly have to do with experimenting. I encourage you to try, try, try. And have fun. That's the most important thing to remember. Please think of me as your cheerleader. *You can do this!* You never know—you may discover gold along the way.

The seven ideas below are quick and straight to the point. I don't want to overwhelm you. The idea is to get you excited, get your creative juices flowing, and inspire you to action. If you're going to take a deeper dive into this strategy, I've listed three additional resources at the end, created by a few of my music therapy colleagues. The seven ideas can be used with any age, population, and type of caregiving; however, my specialization is music in dementia care, so the focus is dementia caregiving.

Let's get into it and take a look at seven ways for you and your loved one to daily experience joy and connection through music:

SING

Did you know singing has a ton of health benefits? In many ways, singing is similar to exercise. Because it's an aerobic activity, it gets more oxygen into the blood, leading to better circulation, which can cause improved mood. Singing causes the release of endorphins, which gives us that wonderful "lifted" feeling, often resulting in stress relief. Best of all, because singing requires deep breathing, a natural result is often reduced anxiety.

Even if you don't describe yourself as a singer, know that everyone has a voice, and you can use your voice to sing! The cool thing about your voice is it's an instrument that is always with you anywhere you go. It's as simple as turning on a song and singing along. Create a playlist of you and your loved one's favorite tunes to sing together. (Take advantage of free or low-cost resources like YouTube or Spotify.) Learn the lyrics of a few songs together so you can sing a cappella (voice only) when you can't conveniently turn on music. A few more ideas for you and your loved one to regularly sing include: participating in a choir together, trying karaoke, taking voice lessons, or receiving music therapy services.

PLAY

Instrument play is fun and can provide playfulness, self-expression, and physical movement opportunities. You can play musical instruments alone or with accompaniment music. Do you or your loved one own any musical instruments? It's time to pull them out. Play for fun—don't worry about how you sound or if you're playing correctly. You don't necessarily need to know how to play. Start by exploring the instrument and see what sounds you can make.

Small, shakeable percussion instruments like maracas are generally easy to pick up and play without previous knowledge or experience. Turn on some music and have fun jamming out with your instruments. Here are some additional instrument ideas to get you thinking: harmonica, hand drums, tambourine, jingle bells, egg shakers, paddle drums, buffalo drums, or ukulele. I recommend a Studio 49 Easycussion pentatonic xylophone, Suzuki Q-Chord, or a Remo ocean drum for a few unique instrument options. Visit https://www.westmusic.com for quality instruments at reasonable prices.

DANCE

We are rhythmic beings. Music is a natural motivator for the physical body. Adding rhythm to movement is often an automatic response when we hear music. We often tap our toes or bob our heads to the beat, sometimes without even thinking! Dance and movement are the body's natural response to rhythm. So, turn on some music and just dance!

Choosing familiar or well-known songs can be helpful, but don't shy away from exploring new-to-you and different types of music. You never know what new songs or styles you'll discover. To help get you thinking, here are some genres of music to which you could dance: big band, jazz, rock'n'roll, folk, bluegrass, country/western, classical, rhythm and blues, gospel, pop, Broadway show tunes, soul, funk, and disco.

You can try formal dances like the waltz, tango, or cha-cha-cha or make your own moves. Try embracing and swaying to the music together or facing each other and doing seated movement to the music. Try stretching, exercising, or doing body percussion, which uses your body to create a rhythmic beat. Try clapping your hands, snapping your fingers, patting your lap or chest, stomping your feet, kicking, tapping, marching, shaking, waving, etc. Get creative!

LISTEN

Listening to music can be an enjoyable activity all on its own. Find a playlist you and your loved one enjoy, or create your own. Listening to music is an excellent activity for relaxation or brain stimulation. It can be a passive, receptive experience by simply listening. Or, it can be an active, engaging experience by discussing the lyrics and various elements of the music, such as the sound, feel, different instruments involved, etc. There is no right or wrong way to listen to music. Do what feels best and what you both enjoy most.

Listening to music also accompanies other activities, such as cleaning, cooking, running errands, or doing an art project. One word of caution: Beware of over-stimulation when using music this way. Many activities require a great amount of focus, and some types of music can lead to the brain having too much to process at once. Try to match the musical energy to the energy level of your activity. Instrumental (music without lyrics) can work well when you and your loved one need to talk during an activity. Music can also be an amazing catalyst for reminiscence. To start, choose songs associated with positive, meaningful memories. Observe your loved one as you listen together, and consider asking a couple of questions about the song afterward.

RELAX

Music can be a wonderful tool for relaxation. The music I find calming may differ from the music you find calming, so you need to consider and choose calming music for you and your loved one. There is some overlap between listening to music and relaxing to music. Turn on relaxing music during a calming, creative activity like painting or coloring. Try also using music as a structured space for deep breathing, gentle stretching, intentional relaxation, or meditation. There're different techniques for each of these, but don't get bogged down in the how-to. Begin by experimenting to see what it's like using music to assist in relaxation, then go from there. If you're at a loss as to what kind of music to play for intentional relaxation, try looking up a playlist of the type of music spas use during massage therapy and other treatments. Nature soundscapes or ambient music can work beautifully to calm the mind and body.

WRITE

Creating a song can be a fun, expressive activity for anyone and a beautiful way to connect with your loved one. Songwriting is sometimes a multi-step process involving several layers: choosing a song structure, writing lyrics, composing a melody, and creating harmony or accompaniment. However, you don't need to be a musician to write a song, so don't be intimidated by this activity. It can be as simple as making up a short melody to hum, writing some lyrics, or taking a preexisting song and replacing the words with your own (known as a song parody).

Don't worry about music theory, song structure, chord progressions, or any other technical formalities with songwriting. Allow your creative juices to flow! Be sure to record your song somehow—write it down or record a quick voice memo. You could also write a formal full-length song with your loved one. This could take place over the span of a few hours or over a few weeks or months as an ongoing project. If one or both of you play an instrument, that'll help create the melody and chords.

RECORD

This is a reminder to capture all those moments of joy and connection that result from making music together. Use the voice memo app on your phone or your phone's camera to record a video. Write down special moments in a notebook. Capture these meaningful musical moments in some way. You'll be grateful later on. To take it a step further, share with friends and family. They'll appreciate it, and those special, memorable moments will become even more so.

A FEW TIPS

These tips may help you push past any initial discomfort or unfamiliarity:

- **Keep it simple.** I want you to remember this tip. Don't feel like what you try needs to be a performance. We, as humans, excel at over-complicating things. KISS (keep it simple, silly).

- **Give yourself permission.** Be willing to experiment, to fail, and even to feel a little silly in the process. Don't be self-conscious about how you look or sound. If you struggle to permit yourself to try something outside your comfort zone, I hereby grant you full permission to make music! Don't shy away from doing something simply because you've never done it before.

- **Something is always worth trying.** You never know what gold you may discover along the way. You're trying something that could lead to an incredible, positive outcome, so don't knock it 'til you try it.

- **Become a detective.** What are your loved one's musical preferences? Do a little digging to discover what kinds of music or music activities they resonate with most. Ask other family members and close friends of your loved one what specific songs, genres, styles, and musical artists they enjoy. This can make all the difference. If you can't glean many specifics, employ a trial-and-error approach, noting how they respond.

- **Start somewhere.** If incorporating a music-based activity into your daily routine is overwhelming at first, start small. Try weekly or monthly.

- **Have fun!** The most important thing to remember when incorporating music into dementia caregiving is to have fun! Music is a gift. It can be a beautiful catalyst for sparking joy and connection. Remember, music is powerful. Like a vitamin, a little bit every day nourishes the heart, mind, and soul.

QUICK LIST OF IDEAS TO GET YOU GOING

- Join a community choir or specialized dementia choir
- Attend concerts
- Try karaoke
- Play an instrument
- Seek out a music therapist
- Listen to music every day
- Ask questions about the song lyrics
- Find dementia-friendly music programs
- Create a personalized playlist
- Feel the rhythm: Move to music
- Make up dance moves
- Play musical games such as "Name that tune"
- Use body percussion
- Relax to music
- Write a song
- Record musical moments

ADDITIONAL RESOURCES FOR A DEEPER DIVE

Listen, Sing, Dance, Play: Bring Musical Moments into the Rhythms of Caregiving by Rachelle Morgan

Music, Memory, and Meaning: How to Effectively Use Music to Connect with Aging Loved Ones by Meredith Hamons, Tara Jenkins and Cathy Befi-Hensel

Musically Engaged Seniors: 40 Session Plans and Resources for a Vibrant Music Therapy Program by Meredith Hamons

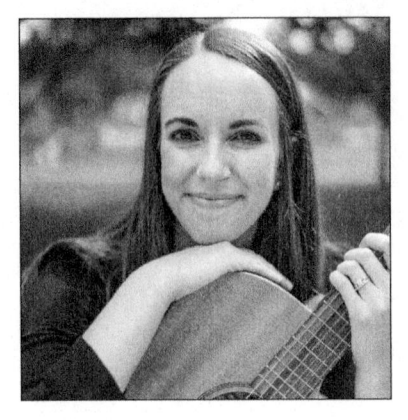

Alexis Baker is a board-certified music therapist (MT-BC), certified dementia practitioner (CDP), and founder of Bridgetown Music Therapy. Her mission as a music therapist is to spark joy and improve quality of life through meaningful music engagement. Alexis is passionate about using music to make a difference in the lives of older adults living with dementia and their caregivers.

After years spent serving clients in person as a traveling music therapist, Alexis pivoted her business online in 2020. In response to the Covid-19 pandemic, she and her husband, a professional videographer, decided to collaborate by putting their skills together. They launched a virtual music engagement program with a robust Member Library containing hundreds of videos on demand. Their dementia-friendly music sessions focus on meaningful engagement through music-based activities such as singing, gentle stretching and movement, deep breathing exercises, and relaxation. Alexis includes an incredible range of genres, styles, and fun themes—there is something for everyone. This program has been described as a *game-changer for people* with dementia and their caregivers.

A few of Alexis' favorite things, in no particular order, are sunflowers, coffee, the beach, dark chocolate, essential oils, travel, outdoor adventures, inspirational quotes, and reading. Outside of her business, she and her husband run an international nonprofit called 501 Collective. Alexis loves Jesus, her husband, her family, and helping others.

Connect with Alexis:

Website: https://www.bridgetownmt.com or email: Alexis@BridgetownMT.com

LinkedIn: https://www.linkedin.com/in/alexisbaker-mt-bc/

Facebook: https://www.facebook.com/bridgetownmusictherapy

Instagram: https://www.instagram.com/bridgetownmusictherapy/

YouTube: https://www.youtube.com/@bridgetownmt

CHAPTER 2

When It's Time for the Talk

TURN AWKWARD CONVERSATIONS INTO ACTIONABLE ELDERCARE PLANNING

Amy Friesen, Business and Caregiver Coach

MY STORY

My husband and I crowded around my desk as we dialed his dad's phone number, placed the phone on the desk, and pressed speaker. "How are you, Dad? What's new?" I could see him working up the courage to broach the sensitive topic of Dad coming to live with us.

His dad's health was failing, and he lived eight hours away from us with no other family around. Additionally, we wanted to see him more. COVID was difficult on all of us, and we hadn't seen him for two years, which meant he also never got to see his only granddaughter, who was four at the time. We tossed bits and pieces of this conversation out over the last few years, none of which seemed to stick.

I watched my husband wring his hands and stutter while he tried not once but twice to bring up a conversation with his dad that was already a topic of conversation in our house for the last year. He looked over at me as if asking for help, and I had to decide whether I'd be stepping on toes if I stepped in, or if my professional background would now come in handy. I whispered to him, "Do you want me to jump in?" he nodded in agreement.

"Dad," I said. "Mike and I have been talking about it, and we would really love to see more of you and for you to be able to be with Eva. I know things have been tough this last while, and we feel that if you moved in with us, not only could we help, but you could also be around family." And with that, a totally unexpected pause. I heard the wheels turning while he considered, but he didn't need any extra time to think it over this time. "Okay, let's do it." I looked over at Mike. He looked at me with a sigh of relief; his whole body relaxed. We had finally gotten there, and a huge looming burden of stress lifted like hundreds of pounds dropping from our shoulders.

You know that feeling you get in your stomach when there are some large, life-changing decisions about to be made, but you don't feel like you have enough information, experience, or communication about what you're deciding on? Families of seniors have this feeling all day long, and it can last weeks, months, and sometimes even years. Complications in the health system, unknown housing options, stubborn loved ones, and adult children not wanting to have awkward conversations make for an emotionally charged, confusing journey through eldercare.

For two decades, I've worked with families at all stages of the journey, including individuals who didn't want to move from their homes to seniors ready to go and move into retirement living with all the bells and whistles. Although there are many reasons and objections, the number one stumbling block I see is individuals not wanting to have awkward conversations.

I've had adult children tell me every day, "I don't want to have that conversation." Or "Can't I just tell Mom she smells?" Or even "We'll just deal with things when something happens." Every day, I think to myself, *man, eldercare conversations are so awkward for these families.*

Here's an example. You show up to pick Mom up for groceries and smell something funny. Her house seems to smell like pee all of a sudden. You give Mom a once over and notice her clothing is clean and her hair is brushed, but you can't help but notice a strong odor. You're embarrassed for yourself and her and think *I can't bring her grocery shopping like this, but how do I tell her she smells? She must be able to smell the same thing I can.*

In this situation, there could be many reasons that Mom isn't addressing the odor. She may not be able to smell it as strongly or at all. She may have some cognitive decline, or she may just be embarrassed and not want to ask for help. It's time for an awkward conversation for all these reasons and more.

Beyond the "Birds and the Bees" conversation, you might have thought you'd escaped it all. However, as adults, new discussions arise akin to something I refer to as "The Talks of Eldercare." These are often more difficult conversations that center around obtaining accurate information, safety awareness, making informed decisions, and ensuring everyone is on the same page. Ultimately, these discussions equip families with the necessary resources to successfully navigate the complexities of the eldercare journey.

But why are "The Talks" so tough? There are several reasons why these conversations feel more difficult. Carving out the time and coordinating schedules alone is a challenge. This is especially difficult when you're trying to schedule something you don't want to do or trying to schedule with a loved one who's in a bit of denial. Additionally, like many other pieces of the eldercare journey, these conversations are most likely things you've had no training for and no prior experience with. The pure heaviness of "The Talks" means many families avoid having them and usually find themselves dangerously close to or in a crisis.

Have you ever heard the saying "steer into the skid"? In other words, look where you're going in order to have better control of what lies ahead of you. In my 20 years, I've encountered a very small percentage of proactive families. Unfortunately, many families I speak with are already in a health crisis.

A health crisis is an emotionally charged and fast-paced situation where families often need to make quick decisions based on limited information. A crisis means all hands on deck. There are often many moving parts in these situations; they need to be coordinated, and families also need to create a strategy.

EMOTIONAL ASPECTS OF AN IMPENDING HEALTH CRISIS

As a health crisis begins to emerge, there are a series of emotional stages and experiences individuals go through when they're coping with loss or significant life changes. They include:

1. **Denial** of needing help on the part of both the senior and the caregiver.
2. **Anger and stress** from needing to deal with a situation you'd rather not have to deal with.
3. **Bargaining** for ways to remain in the familiar situation.
4. **Grief** is the emotional process of mourning and adjusting to losses associated with aging, declining health, and eventual death of self/loved ones.
5. **Depression and overwhelm** from having a lot to do and not knowing where to start.
6. **Acceptance**—safety outweighs familiar comfort, and a transition is made.

However, there's a way to lessen the effects of changing health—crisis can be mitigated. There are huge benefits to being proactive in eldercare planning. The top benefits of planning are choice and control. You may say, "Amy, I don't feel in control of my circumstances." While this feeling is true of many people, you have substantially more control over how you and your loved ones' life plays out on the eldercare journey if you make room for awkward conversations and start them sooner rather than later.

THE STRATEGY

How to set up "The Talk" for success.

The purpose of having these seven talks is to set up a care path. I define care path planning as a comprehensive strategy that anticipates various healthcare scenarios, ensuring corresponding plans are prepared and accessible when needed. Another key characteristic of a carepath plan is that it's reviewed regularly and adapted to changing circumstances.

The 7 Talks of Eldercare that will assist you in creating a personalized care path plan are:

1. **The Financial Talk**

    Serves multiple purposes, primarily focusing on budgeting, adapting to changes in living situations, and facilitating access to funds.

2. **The Expectation Talk**

    Revolves around crucial aspects such as caregiver time, financial considerations, and the dynamics of caregiving.

3. **The Mental Health Talk**

    Tackles a spectrum of critical facets, encompassing discussions on dementia diagnosis, depression, anxiety, isolation, and medication management.

4. **The Physical Health Talk**

    Centers on various aspects, including identifying the individuals involved in providing physical care, determining the timing and frequency of their assistance, and outlining specific care needs.

5. **The Living Arrangements Talk**

    Delves into various critical aspects, focusing on priorities, timelines for relocation, destination considerations, underlying reasons, and financial implications, including costs and benefits.

6. **The Legal Talk**

    Revolves around essential legal documents, including powers of attorney, advance directives and wills.

7. **The End of Life Talk**

    This is a deeply important conversation centered on preparedness, encompassing discussions about completed arrangements, the organization of important documents and belongings, and the articulation of personal preferences.

Most heavy conversations in eldercare will fall under one of the above talks. Some could be easier than others depending on the family dynamic, communication styles, and timing, while others will be more difficult.

Below, you'll find tips on how to have some of these conversations within the family so you can create a carepath that works for everyone involved. Every difficult conversation must have a few fundamental things to be successful.

"THE TALK" MUST HAVE'S

- Acknowledgement of the difficult conversation and situation
- The right time and the right place
- Involvement of all key family members
- Active listening and reading body language
- Open, non-judgemental communication
- Follow-up steps

ACKNOWLEDGEMENT OF THE DIFFICULT CONVERSATION AND SITUATION

Sometimes, saying "This is a difficult conversation" to the other person helps to put them at ease and opens the door for discussion. If both the adult child and the senior are struggling with having the conversation and sharing that knowledge with each other, the situation will begin to look less like a struggle and more like a collaboration. Expressing that these types of talks are uncomfortable and mapping out an easier way to have them will lighten the mood. Don't be afraid to use some humor as well. Acknowledging the awkwardness might just be the trick.

What my mom said to my dad when he hurt his hand and couldn't use it for a number of months:

"I know that you're struggling with this setback even though you don't show it. I know it's difficult for you to talk to me about it, and things are hard when you won't be able to use your right hand for a little bit. We'll figure it out, and I'm happy to help with anything you need, but let's get a bidet because I'm not wiping your butt!"

THE RIGHT TIME AND THE RIGHT PLACE

No one wants an uncomfortable conversation thrust upon them. Most want time to consider the subject matter and compile their thoughts. Additionally, it's important to make sure that "The Talk" has been prearranged and happens in an appropriate setting. This will give your family the best chance at success to get these conversations out in the open. The scene can be set like this:

"Mom, I'm coming over for lunch tomorrow at noon, and I was hoping we could discuss my concerns about your bad knees and the number of steps in your home to see if we can come up with some better solutions."

INVOLVEMENT OF ALL KEY FAMILY MEMBERS

Making sure you have the buy-in of all your key family members might seem like an unnecessary step, but most of the conversations in eldercare have a range of opinions attached to them. Because of this, informing the other family members of the upcoming conversations and involving them will often go a long way toward preventing obstacles when one family member is not on board.

Nothing is worse than settling on decisions and a plan of action and then having a sibling who hasn't been involved jump in and offer "their two cents." Even as a professional, I see this happen all the time. When this happens, the person just surfacing usually says something like, "I think mom is fine at home." Meanwhile, they're not the primary caregiver, nor do they realize how difficult and time-consuming this decision has been. Additionally, once that statement is out there, it opens the doubt door and pauses the momentum.

"I don't think we need to move. I can still do the stairs. Besides, Jon thinks I am fine here."

It's best to ensure everyone is on the same page before this type of conversation happens with your loved one(s) to reduce the conflict between family members and the probability of a backslide.

ACTIVE LISTENING AND READING BODY LANGUAGE

I often tell families it's not only active listening but also reading body language that's important. Not everyone knows how to express themselves, and often, a lot is unsaid. This is especially true of someone who has cognitive decline. If you can pick up on non-verbal clues and feelings that were not said, you can add some open-ended questions to suss out what the real objections are. We all have fears about aging, and adult children have their own fears and worry about their senior loved ones. These conversations can be difficult on everyone, so watching for the unsaid is just as important as the said.

"What I hear you saying is that this has been your home for 50 years, and the thought of leaving it is overwhelming and makes you sad. Is that right?"

OPEN, NON-JUDGEMENTAL COMMUNICATION

These types of talks should be a judgment-free zone. You're asking your loved one to share things that might be their biggest fears and share them with their children. Parents spend a lifetime trying to shield their children from harmful or stressful situations. It will be important to communicate with your loved one that you're there to help and share mutual goals.

"Mom, I know it's difficult to talk about this sensitive topic. Rest assured that there are no judgments on my end. I only want to help you remain safe and cared for. That is what is most important to me."

SETTING FOLLOW-UP STEPS

A plan without action is a dream. Following up, re-evaluating, and tweaking are all a part of the planning process. No one's life stays the same forever, and there may be small tweaks you can make along the way to keep things on track, but unless you regularly look at the plan, you won't know. Worse yet, you may accidentally go off plan in as easy as one decision and create an entire situation you didn't want. Schedule regular touch points as a family to review the plan and decide if it still works or needs to be tweaked.

It's often difficult for individuals to reach out for help and they often feel very alone in their situation. I can tell you that you're not alone. Many families are moving through the eldercare journey just as you are. What's really interesting to see as a professional is that a few core situations vary only in small details. These talks will help you address the main issues in eldercare and ensure your family is on the best and safest path moving forward. Remember, reaching out for support is a crucial step towards ensuring the well-being of your loved ones and yourself.

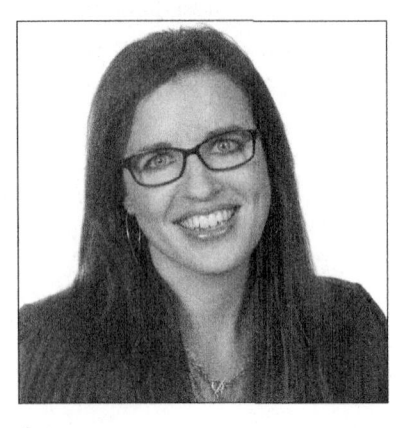

Amy Friesen is widely recognized as a luminary in the field of senior living and is celebrated for her diverse roles as a best-selling author, educator, and expert. In 2014, driven by a profound dedication to enriching the lives of seniors and their families worldwide, Amy founded Tea & Toast in 2014, a pioneering initiative aimed at providing invaluable support in navigating the complexities of housing and healthcare for seniors.

Tea & Toast is a testament to Amy's unyielding commitment to fostering better choices and alleviating the often overwhelming burdens associated with eldercare. Her holistic approach to client care not only prioritizes their immediate well-being but also facilitates seamless transitions throughout the eldercare journey, infused with compassion, empathy, and seasoned expertise.

The unique methodology employed by Tea & Toast has become a beacon of hope for countless families, offering personalized assistance tailored to individual needs and aspirations. By meticulously planning for short and long-term goals, Amy and her team alleviate the stressors inherent in eldercare, allowing families to navigate this pivotal phase with confidence and peace of mind.

In addition to her groundbreaking work with Tea & Toast, Amy is the visionary behind a cross-Canada association of Eldercare Planning Professionals, advocating for caregiver support, senior living, and comprehensive aging solutions. Amy's leadership in the senior housing industry has earned her widespread recognition, including the prestigious 2018 Businesswoman of the Year Award acknowledged by the House of Commons and a recipient of the 2019 Forty Under 40 award.

Amy's influence extends far beyond her professional accolades, permeating various media platforms where she has been featured in numerous news interviews and sought-after as a guest on podcasts. Through these channels, she generously shares her wealth of knowledge and insights on senior living and eldercare planning, enriching discourse and understanding.

For more information, please visit:

https://www.teaandtoast.ca

https://www.teaandtoast.ca/the-talk

https://www.amyfriesen.com

https://www.eldercareplanning.ca

CHAPTER 3

Building Your Support Team

THE ART AND FREEDOM OF ASKING FOR AND ACCEPTING HELP

Cheryl M. Kinney, MSW, LCSW

MY STORY

Why do those who give so much often have so much trouble asking for and accepting help from others?

That thought came to mind when Mary arrived for our dementia coaching session and burst into tears the moment the door to my office closed. Her hands shook as she described her daily struggle to take over things her husband Bill always handled before Alzheimer's began robbing him of his memories and his ability to do even simple tasks at home.

I knew that look of hopeless defeat in her tear-swollen, red-rimmed eyes after spending years guiding thousands just like her through the challenges of caregiving.

Mary began telling me her story.

"I spent the last three days trying to balance the checkbook. Bill was an accountant so he always handled all the money stuff. I never even looked at a bank statement. Last week we got letters from the gas and water companies saying they're going to cut off our service. He wasn't paying the bills! I have no idea what I'm doing."

Like many other care partners, Mary was suddenly faced with having to take on tasks she was unprepared to handle. And it wasn't just the household bill-paying responsibility she now had to take over.

"He lost his driver's license after he had several accidents. Now, he wants me to drive him to the golf course every day. It's winter! No one plays golf when it's snowing out! I don't like to drive on a good weather day."

Mary's hands were clenched tightly in her lap as though she had a steel grip on the steering wheel while trying to navigate through a snowstorm.

In addition to taking on things at home that Bill always handled, she was now facing behaviors that further added to her stress.

"He gets up in the middle of the night and says he needs to get to work. He's been retired for ten years! I have to beg him to get back in bed. He looks at me like he doesn't know me!"

It's obvious that Mary isn't getting enough sleep.

"Last night, the smoke alarm started going off at 3 a.m., and Bill just stared at it. I had no idea what to do. I finally just threw a shoe at it! I'm at my wit's end."

Yup. Overwhelmed. Exhausted. Defeated.

I didn't have to tell Mary that providing care and support can put a tremendous physical, financial, emotional, and spiritual toll on the caregiver. She was deep in the throes of it, and the circles under her red-rimmed eyes made it obvious that she was stressed to the limit.

And now her health was affected. Her doctor referred her to me because her blood pressure had reached a dangerously high level.

She's so stressed out she's going to end up having a stroke if things don't improve soon. Then who's going to care for Bill?

As Mary's story unfolded, I learned more about her family and friends. She and Bill have a daughter and son who live nearby. Bill has a group of guys he used to work with that he gets together with every week for coffee. Many of their neighbors and people from their church are considered their closest friends.

When we began talking about which of these people she feels comfortable turning to for support, she responded with those words I've heard so often through the years:

"Oh, I would never ask for help."

"I don't want to be a burden."

"They have so much going on in their own lives."

I bet Mary would be the first person in line to help each of these people, but she can't bring herself to ask the same of them in return.

I get it. I'm just like Mary. I've been there too.

My husband, Jack, has received treatment for cancer off and on for the past 15 years. While he has responded well to the chemo, the side effects have been rough at times. I've felt the stress of trying to juggle work and home responsibilities while watching him grow so weak he could barely walk across the room. I've hidden my tears after coming home from work to find that he hadn't eaten all day.

When he was in the hospital for five weeks for a stem cell transplant, he hated the hospital food. So, after a long day of work, I would pick up dinner from a local restaurant for the two of us to eat, then spend an hour or so with him. By the time I got home, all I wanted to do was crawl in bed. But there was a dog to walk and papers to grade for the class I was teaching.

Fortunately, we've been blessed with plenty of offers of help, support, and prayers.

"Let me know how I can help."

"Do you want me to take the dog for a walk?"

"Can I bring Jack dinner so you can take a night off?"

I'd like to say I always accepted the offers of help. But honestly, I've been guilty of trying to convince myself I'm strong and able to handle anything that's put on my plate.

I've learned through experience that doing so only leads us down a very dark and lonely road.

Because I've traveled a similar journey as Mary and many others like her, I've made it a personal mission to help the caregivers I work with accept that trying to do everything on our own isn't best for us or the person we're caring for.

I gently told Mary the importance of taking care of herself so that she could be the best support possible for Bill.

"Mary, this is something no one can, or should, do on their own. If you get sick, you won't be there for Bill. Let's talk about how you can begin to lighten your load."

Together, we moved into the problem-solving stage of our session by identifying her immediate needs, looking toward possible future needs, and then talking about how informal and formal support providers may meet these needs. We even role-played how she might respond to offers from family and friends and how to overcome her reluctance to ask for help.

I could see the tension slowly leaving Mary's body as she worked to create a plan for turning some of Bill's care and their household responsibilities over to others.

Mary reached out to hug me as she left my office. "Thank you so much. I can see now that I'm not alone."

Now it's your turn. I'll teach you some simple steps to build your support team and increase your confidence in asking for and accepting help.

THE STRATEGY

STEP 1: LEARN TO ASK FOR AND ACCEPT HELP

Learning to ask for and accept help is an art. And much like learning to paint and sculpt, you will feel more confident over time as you start practicing this art. Once you get the hang of it, you'll feel a sense of freedom when you let go and let others share the responsibility of supporting the care receiver.

The first step in building a support team is acknowledging that you need help. This is followed by giving yourself the freedom to ask for and accept that help.

As humans, we're naturally wired to avoid appearing weak. Going back to the beginning of time, being weak made us vulnerable to injury, illness, and prey. But instead of thinking that asking for help is a sign of weakness, think of it as a sign of strength: seeking support is a proactive step we can take toward caring for ourselves and others.

> *"Alone, we can do so little; together we can do so much."*
>
> ~ Helen Keller

In the Christian faith and many other faiths, we're called to serve others. The Bible teaches us to "Bear one another's burdens, and so fulfill the law of Christ" (Galatians 6:2). Therefore, when you allow someone else to give the gift of helping you in your time of need, you're allowing them to serve God.

Scottish author Alexander McCall Smith said it this way: "Gracious acceptance is an art - an art which most never bother to cultivate. We think that we have to learn how to give, but we forget about accepting things, which can be much harder than giving. Accepting another person's gift is allowing him to express his feelings for you."

Think about how you may be keeping someone else from having the opportunity to spend time with the care receiver by not including them as part of that person's support team.

Mary told me she didn't want to bother her son and daughter.

"They are so busy with their own lives."

She would tell them everything was okay when they called or stopped by. She never mentioned how little sleep she was getting. She made up excuses when her son asked about the new dents in the fender of Bill's car.

Mary told me how her daughter Karen had always idolized her dad and how she even became an accountant herself to follow in his footsteps.

"I don't want her to see her dad this way. Sometimes, he even forgets her name."

I explained to Mary that because Bill has a progressive disease, there will come a time when he won't be able to talk with Karen. But right now, it means a lot to him when she tells him how her new job is going.

Suddenly, it became clear to her:

"I've been trying so hard to protect them from all this that I've kept them from spending time with their dad."

DON'T SAY "NO"

Receiving help reminds us that we're not alone. But sometimes the help someone offers isn't what we need at the time.

Just like the neon-colored fuzzy slippers your Aunt Mildred gave you for your birthday that were two sizes too small, some gifts aren't the right size or style for you. That's okay. If someone offers to help in a way that isn't needed at the time, don't decline the help. Instead, "exchange it" for something you do need.

Mary started building her confidence in accepting help by turning an offer that didn't quite fit into something that would bring some much-needed relief.

"Bill's friend offered to stay with him so I could go out to lunch. I told him what would really help would be for him to bring Bill home after the men's coffee on Wednesdays."

His friend was happy to do this and offered to swing by to get Bill on the way to the coffee shop so Mary wouldn't have to drive at all on those days.

DON'T ACCEPT "NO"

Likewise, get in the habit of not accepting "no" for an answer.

When Mary asked her son Brad if he'd come over on Saturday to hang out with Bill so she could run to the store, Brad told her he had to take his daughter to her soccer match. Rather than accepting "no," Mary practiced her new-found skill of asking for help.

"I started to ask if he could pick up a few things for me from the grocery store on his way home from the game, but then I got the idea to ask him if he would take his dad with him to Maddy's game so I could go to the store myself!"

Brad loved the idea.

"He couldn't wait to tell me how excited his dad got when Maddy waved to him from the field. He even got to see her score her first goal!" "Bill talked about that game for a whole week!"

It was a win for everyone!

STEP 2: LIST CURRENT AND FUTURE NEEDS

It's best to have a mental list of things others can do to help so you are ready when an offer is made. Better still, put it in writing!

Start by drawing a line down the middle of a lined piece of paper.

On the left side, write down all the things you can think of that you could delegate to others. The sky is the limit here. There's no judgment. If you want to delegate cleaning the cat's litter box, write it down!

If the need is urgent or time-specific, include a note stating when the task needs to be done.

Mary got her son and daughter to help start her list. The first draft included things she needed help with right away and some things she would need help with in the future:

- Rides to the men's coffee group
- Sign up for online bill-paying
- Buy and install a new smoke alarm (this week)
- Lawn mowing (spring-summer)
- Get someone to file the taxes (April)
- Research care options: in-home care, adult day services, long-term care

STEP 3: IDENTIFY INFORMAL AND FORMAL (PROFESSIONAL) SUPPORT

On the right side of the paper, list all the people and resources that could meet each need. If you only think of one person or resource that can help, try to identify a backup if that person isn't available.

First, list potential informal support team members:

- Family
- Friends
- Neighbors
- Faith community members

You might feel more comfortable starting with those who have already offered to help in some way.

Next, fill in the list with formal (professional) support services:

- Doctors, nurses, and other healthcare professionals
- In-home care agencies and other formal care providers
- Nutrition, food, and meal services
- Area agencies on aging
- Handyman services

Social workers and care managers can answer questions about care options and funding sources that may pay for care, such as Medicare, Medicaid, the Veterans Administration, and community grants.

Voluntary health organizations such as the Alzheimer's Association, the American Parkinson's Disease Association, and the American Cancer Society can help caregivers know what to expect in the future. Many have online resources and toll-free helplines to answer questions and provide disease-specific information.

Elder law attorneys can create necessary legal documents such as a durable power of attorney and advance directives.

Financial advisors can assist in determining the funds the care recipient has available to pay for the care that may be required and ways to avoid financial exploitation. (See Chapter 8: The Art of Financial Self-Defense).

STEP 4: FINE-TUNE YOUR LIST

Think of the list you create as a work in progress. Your first draft will be messy. Take your time and add things as they come to mind. Ask others to help create the list (flex that new "asking for help" muscle!).

After you capture as many needs and resources as possible, transfer the information to a more permanent document. Add to it and adjust the list as needs change.

OVERCOMING RESISTANCE AND MANAGING EXPECTATIONS

As mentioned before, the art of asking for help must be developed over time. Some caregivers have no trouble delegating responsibility. Others may find themselves "yes, butting" at the very thought. If you found yourself thinking of why you can't turn tasks and responsibilities over to others while reading this chapter, you're not alone!

Here is how Mary responded when I introduced the idea of having a friend or an in-home companion stay with Bill so she could go to the beauty shop once a week:

"Yes, but Bill would never agree to have someone 'babysit' him!"

I suggested she ask her daughter or one of Bill's friends to take him to lunch on the day of her appointment.

"He'll enjoy the outing, and you'll be glad not to have him tell you how to drive the whole way to your hair appointment!"

Sometimes, just looking at the situation from another perspective will help you embrace the freedom of asking for and accepting help.

It's important to consider who you can trust and rely on to help. This means managing your expectations. If you haven't had contact with your daughter for ten years, it's best not to assume she will be there for you if you call. If your neighbor keeps telling you how busy they are when you ask for help, cross them off your list.

One caregiver I worked with told me that her son made it clear to her that he was never going to change his dad's diapers. While this was hard for her to accept, she agreed it was better to know this upfront so she wouldn't be disappointed if the situation ever arose. Instead, we talked about home care agencies that could assist as needed. After our consultation, she sat down with her son, and they came up with other ways he could help, like running errands and mowing the grass.

If you're struggling with the concept of sharing your care responsibilities, start by accepting a few offers (or exchanging them for something that works best for you). Then, ease into asking for a small favor.

Consider talking to a social worker or therapist for help in working through the barriers to letting go.

Remember: Receiving help is a gift you give to the person who helps you and a gift you give yourself. There is freedom in sharing the care you are providing with others. Know that you are not alone!

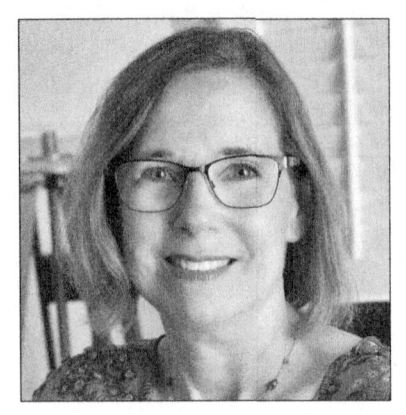

Cheryl M. Kinney, MSW, is a licensed clinical social worker, certified life coach, private therapist, and former instructor of university-level classes on aging and dementia with over 35 years of experience guiding older adults and caregivers using a disease-management approach. In 2017, she was awarded the Washington University Center on Aging Harvey A. and Dorismae Hacker Freidman Award for excellence in service to older adults.

Her professional work with those impacted by dementia and her personal experience supporting her father and other family members through their journey with Alzheimer's have driven Cheryl's mission to change the course of the disease. In 2020, Cheryl co-founded Memory Keepers, a modified version of cognitive stimulation therapy for those with mild to moderate dementia. Cheryl and business partner Britt Lueken offer weekly classes designed to improve mood, cognition, and quality of life. In 2023, Memory Keepers was launched as a packaged subscription-based program now used by those in the aging and dementia care field in multiple states. A Caregiver Support program package was added in 2024.

When Cheryl isn't working to change the lives of those impacted by dementia, she can be found reading mystery novels, walking Finnegan, her adorable Wheaton Terrier, cheering on the Missouri Tiger's football team with her husband and biggest cheerleader Jack, or traveling to Texas to visit her amazing daughter and son-in-law.

Connect with Cheryl:

Website: https://www.memorykeepers.org

Facebook: https://www.facebook.com/memorykeepersllc

LinkedIn: https://www.linkedin.com/in/cheryl-kinney-42822688/

Instagram: https://www.instagram.com/memorykeepersllc/

CHAPTER 4

Be Their Power

LEGAL DOCUMENTS ALL CAREGIVERS NEED

Karen Hulme Alegi, Attorney

MY STORY

Sitting in my office on a sunny afternoon, my phone buzzes, and the office admin says there is a PC (potential client) on the phone and that she wants to get a power of attorney for her mother. "Can you do that?"

"Of course," I respond. "Send the call in." I introduce myself and get the caller's name. We'll call her Penny. Then I ask her mom's full name and to tell me about Mom and the situation. She gives me the following details:

Penny is the oldest of four siblings.

Penny has been taking care of Mom for the last three years.

Penny takes Mom to all of her doctor's appointments.

Penny pays her mom's bills by writing out the checks on Mom's bank account and having Mom sign her name on the check.

Penny talks to Mom's doctors, the pharmacist, the dentist, and the mailman.

Oh, and Penny moved into Mom's house last year so she could keep a better eye on her. This will also help Penny out since she is trying to get back on her feet after her recent divorce. It works out great because Mom has told Penny that she can stay in the house after Mom passes for as long as she needs to. Penny says her siblings are totally cool with this.

Okay, so "Mom does not have any documents in place now? What's going on that prompted you to call me?"

Penny told me she recently stopped by Mom's bank to order more checks on Mom's bank account. The teller would not allow Penny to order the checks on Mom's account. The teller said either Mom had to come in herself to order the checks or Penny could provide a power of attorney signed by Mom, giving Penny authority to manage the bank account for Mom. Penny does not want to drag her mother into the bank to order the checks herself.

So, Penny asks if I can draft a power of attorney for her mom to sign. "First, tell me about Mom's health?"

Mom is in great shape for 75. She walks every day, still gardens sometimes, and helps with dinner. She loves visits from her grandchildren. Oh, but sometimes she forgets what year it is or calls Penny by Mom's sister's name (Aunt Ruth passed six years ago).

Sounds like dementia. "Has she been diagnosed?"

"Well, not officially. The last time she saw the doctor, it wasn't that bad. But she has been getting worse. I've been meaning to make another appointment with the doctor. But in the meantime, I need the power of attorney, or I cannot pay her bills."

Oops. Problem. I do *not* say this out loud.

I tell Penny, "Let's schedule a time for me to come to your house and meet with you and Mom in person. We have a lot to talk about."

Situations like this give me serious heartburn. Being an attorney, I get to help people everyday work out their problems and feel more secure in their lives, businesses, and finances. That is the best part of the job! But sometimes, new clients have gone too long without legal guidance, and now I have to break the news that the "fix" is much more complicated than it needed to be. Had they worked with me or another attorney sooner, they would be in a much better situation. Every time I have that conversation with potential clients, I get another grey hair. I sincerely hope that this book and others will help change the perception that attorneys are professionals that you only contact when something has gone seriously wrong. Your attorney should be a trusted partner in the beginning of your life journey. I strive to be that for my clients!

THE STRATEGY

The situation that Penny finds herself in is all too common for many people caring for their aging parents. Especially when we live with them, we can be slow to notice just how much their memory and comprehension are fading. Often, it's only when they receive a formal diagnosis from their doctor that they realize that the problem is more serious than they thought.

Penny's problem is that since Mom is already suffering from dementia, Mom no longer has the mental capacity to execute a power of attorney. A power of attorney is a legal document that must be signed by the principal, in this case, Mom, while she is healthy and able to fully understand what she's signing. Because this document is very powerful, strict requirements must be met when executing the document. Even if Mom does not yet have an official diagnosis of dementia or other formal cognitive decline condition, Penny definitely knows Mom is showing signs, and now, I know it, too.

Before we go further, it's important to note that the laws regarding powers of attorney and guardianships are state-specific. Our discussion here will be about general processes and recommendations. Of course, you should consult with a local attorney in your area before taking action. I also never recommend using any do-it-yourself online legal websites. These documents are fraught with errors. It'll cost you much more if you get it wrong. Invest in getting assistance from a competent local attorney.

The document that Penny is asking for is a financial power of attorney, also called a *durable* power of attorney. Any person over the age of 18 and mentally competent can sign a power of attorney giving another person, called an agent or attorney-in-fact, the authority to do anything and everything that the person could do with their property. The person giving the power of attorney is called the principal. The authority in the document often includes the power to sell the house, close or open bank accounts, and sign contracts in the name of the principal. These documents can be customized to address a limited number of assets or are very broad. The key component to the power is that all actions must be for the benefit of the principal, not the agent. So long as the agent acts in good faith, the agent does not bear any personal liability for the financial obligations of the principal.

When this power of attorney is executed and used properly, the agent can easily manage and maintain the principal's assets, accounts, and property and even talk to the bank, mortgage company, and any other person on the principal's behalf. Banks and other institutions cannot refuse to accept a power of attorney properly executed under the state law of the place it was signed.

In addition to property and finances, most caregivers are often the liaison between their loved ones and the healthcare system. Under current federal and state laws, healthcare providers aren't permitted to discuss a person's health or medical information with anyone else unless they have that person's written authorization. This limitation equally applies to spouses and adult children. As we have discussed above, once a person is suffering from or showing signs of dementia, that person no longer has the mental capacity to sign an authorization to release information. It's crucial that your loved one put a healthcare power of attorney in place while they are mentally competent.

A healthcare power of attorney can include several provisions. At a minimum, it names an agent with whom your healthcare professionals are permitted to discuss your medical care, also called a HIPAA Waiver. This authorization typically lists a first choice and a backup and can also list "co-agents." For most situations, I rarely recommend co-agents on any power of attorney. I encourage my clients to pick the one person who is most able to make difficult decisions in stressful situations and name that person as the first choice. Only if your first choice is unavailable can your second choice agent be your decision maker. The purpose of naming one person at a time is to give certainty and clarity to your doctors, nurses, and other healthcare professionals when tough decisions must be made for you.

Your healthcare agent will be your treatment decision-maker once you can no longer communicate on your own. Such treatment decisions can include whether or not to have surgery, consent to testing or transfusions, and end-of-life care options. This last piece is called an advance directive. This document was once referred to as a "living will," but that is a terrible misnomer and creates a lot of confusion. So we shall never use that phrase again! Advance directive language has been standardized throughout most states and will list three different end-of-life medical conditions. For each condition, the principal can select one of three treatment options. These range from letting natural death occur, with or without a feeding tube, to using all available medical means to extend life. These statements are then included in your healthcare power of attorney. The purpose is to give as much information about what you want to your decision-maker as possible when they have to make this decision on your behalf. You can imagine how difficult and stressful this situation will be. So you can help make this decision a bit less stressful by telling your agent what you want in advance.

As a caregiver, you want to have your loved one put these two powers of attorney in place well before they need full-time care. Ideally, they'll have these in place well before any progressive medical conditions. Even if their physical health is in decline, as long as their mental capacity is intact, they can execute the powers of attorney.

But what if your loved one is already suffering from mental decline and has no powers of attorney in place? Since they can no longer execute a power of attorney, without some legal authority, you will have difficulty effectively managing their property and healthcare matters. In most situations, your next option is to file a court proceeding to be appointed as the guardian of your loved one. This guardianship proceeding will vary by state but will generally take the following course. As the petitioner, you file a petition for guardianship of the person and property of your loved one. There'll be a hearing to assess the situation and hear from you personally. You'll have to submit physician certifications of your loved one's medical condition that has necessitated the proceeding. If anyone disagrees with what you are asking for, they can file an objection to your petition. It will ultimately be up to the judge whether or not to establish guardianship and who to appoint as guardians. Once appointed, the guardian must file regular accountings to the court so long as the guardianship is in place.

There are two types of court-appointed guardians: guardians of the property and guardians of the person. Guardian of the property functions just like the agent under a financial power of attorney. The guardian of the property has court-appointed authority to manage the property, assets, and person's accounts. The guardian can pay bills, sign checks, and enter into contracts in the person's name. The guardian of the person takes the place of the healthcare power of attorney and is also responsible for the care and custody of the person. A proceeding can be for just one or both of these types of guardianship.

Because this is a court process, even an uncontested or uncomplicated guardianship proceeding can take several months or longer and cost thousands in attorney's fees. In Maryland and many other states, the court appoints an independent attorney to represent your loved one in the case. This independent attorney meets with all parties and provides an opinion on whether the proposed guardianship is needed (or not). If the person subject to the proposed guardianship does not have cash assets, then the petitioner will have to pay the fees of the independent attorney.

Guardianships are not guaranteed to be granted. The court has to determine that no less restrictive means are available to assist the person. Further, if more than one person wishes to act as the guardian, the matter is contested, and a hearing will be held with witnesses and any other relevant evidence. If more than one hearing is needed and the matter becomes contested, the cost and time to resolve the case will be greatly increased.

Due to the cost, time needed, and uncertainty of outcome, a guardianship proceeding is a last resort. The property drafted and executed powers of attorney we discussed will eliminate the need for a guardianship proceeding. You can have all the power you need to effectively and efficiently manage your loved one's care and property with the proper powers of attorney in place.

No matter where you are in your caregiving journey, if your loved one does not currently have powers of attorney in place, make that your number one priority now. Work with a competent local attorney to ensure the documents are drafted correctly to ensure acceptance and prevent anyone from challenging the documents. And get your own powers of attorney in place while you are at it!

If your loved one is already in mental decline and has no powers of attorney in place, begin your guardianship proceeding now. Yes, it's going to cost more money. But the longer you wait to begin the process, the more stressful, expensive, and difficult it will be to get the resolution you need. Include your loved one's doctors, nurses, social worker, and other family members in the process.

Further, I highly recommend reading Chapter 8 in this book, *The Art of Financial Self-Defense*, to learn more about other strategies to protect your finances, liability, and responsibilities that come along with being a caregiver. You must take care of yourself in order to give the best care to others. Do not overlook your own legal and financial health!

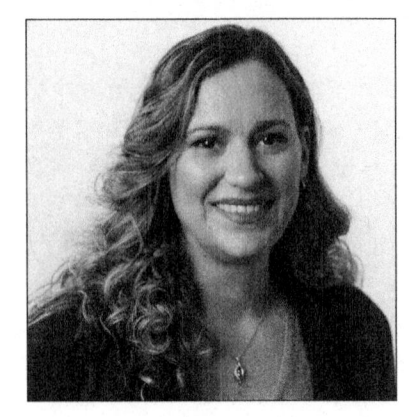

Karen Hulme Alegi, is an attorney in Maryland. She was in private practice for 20 years in which she represented clients in litigation and transactional matters. A significant part of Karen's practice included domestic relations matters, guardianship proceedings, and estate planning. Karen ultimately focused her firm's practice on Wills and Powers of Attorney so that her clients would be prepared for all of life's challenges. Throughout her career, she has strived to educate and inform others about the easy steps everyone can take to protect themselves and their loved ones in declining health, either as a caregiver or one who needs care.

Karen currently works for the Office of Attorney General in Maryland and resides in Gaithersburg with her family. She is active in her local community and enjoys volunteering her time at animal shelters and with organizations that give people second chances. In her free time, you can find her in secondhand stores and antique markets looking for the next treasure!

Connect with Karen

https://www.instagram.com/karenalegiattorney/

https://www.linkedin.com/in/karen-hulme-alegi/

https://alegilaw.com/

CHAPTER 5

Promote Healthy Boundaries to Thrive

CREATE BALANCE FOR RESILIENT AND SUSTAINABLE CAREGIVING

Karen Schuder, EdD, MDiv, MAM

MY STORY

Helping others pulled me into the orbit of their anxiety and emotions, away from the joy I desired. I felt robbed. I wanted to yell, shake my fist, curl into a ball, and cry. I felt as though other people's suffering had blown me off course.

Healthy boundaries were something I needed to learn and that I'll share with you here. There are some practical strategies to promote resilient, sustainable caregiving. You can experience well-being and the joys of your journey while caring for others instead of declining health or burnout.

Caregivers positively change the world. We take on a barrage of demands, such as driving to appointments, filling prescriptions, and cleaning up messes. We share words of encouragement when hope is hard to find. Unexpected hugs and thank yous can make us laugh or cry. We tearfully hold hands with a loved one as they endure pain or take their last breath.

We encounter the best and the worst the world offers while caring for others during difficult times. Despite virtuous efforts, we may have to deal with a family member's criticism or argument about what to do next. Someone's statement communicates, "You didn't do enough," even when we did our best. Love, sorrow, joy, anger, hope, and other emotions fill the caregiving journey.

The emotional mix creates deep meaning as well as exhaustion. We give much of ourselves and discover we have little energy to deal with unexpected problems. Worse yet, our own health declines, so we're unable to take care of others.

CAUGHT IN OTHER PEOPLE'S EMOTIONAL STORMS

Caring about others comes naturally to me but has also come at a cost. During intense caregiver times, heavy demands made it difficult to experience the delights of my own life. One such time was during a Christmas week when responsibilities and exposure to suffering hijacked my hopes for the season.

Christmas lights twinkled, and the scent of pine branches filled my office when I was trying to catch up on work. As a pastor and mother, my to-do list was very long. I spent the beginning of the week sitting with Dori, who was nearing the end of life, listening to Darrel's complaints, and visiting people in care centers. I finally had a chance to tackle the writing I needed to do, but the phone clamored for my attention.

"Hello!" I answered. My greeting was met with gasping sobs.

"I feel so sad and guilty. I can't believe my mom died," said Marcus.

Not again, I thought. Jane died months ago, and this is at least the fourth call. I can't handle another call from him right now.

"Hello, Marcus. I'm sorry to hear you're having a hard time. How can I help you?"

"I don't know. I feel so guilty. I should've done more."

"You gave your mom a wonderful gift of care over the years before she died from cancer at the age of 90. How can I help you find hope and let go of guilt? Can I help you find a grief support group or a therapist?"

"I don't know. I should have done something different."

"Will you please talk to a grief counselor or therapist?"

"I don't know. I don't think it's going to help."

We continued going around these circles for more than an hour. I listened and said encouraging words while my mind wandered.

Christmas time is supposed to be a happy time.

I have so much I need to do.

How can I help him if he won't listen or accept assistance?

Marcus, Dori, Darrel. I feel so powerless and inadequate after these encounters.

"I feel so guilty. I should have done more," repeated Marcus.

"Marcus, I'd be happy to refer you to a therapist or grief counselor when you feel ready. You'll continue to be in my thoughts and prayers. I hope you can find some peace in knowing you gave your mom a wonderful gift and fondly remember her with family this week."

We said goodbyes and a storm cloud settled on my shoulders. I realized that helping others was pulling me into their anxiety and emotions, and away from joy. I learned years ago while providing end-of-life support for my dear mother-in-law that attaching expectations to holiday seasons can be unhelpful. Yet I felt robbed by Marcus and the others.

Rather than walking my path, I was getting pulled into other people's experiences and expectations. I forgot to take responsibility for my own emotions. Previously, I tried to ignore or outrun the effect of other people's suffering, but I learned that this was exhausting.

So, I stopped and looked at the storm. I shed tears and hugged myself. I allowed myself to release other people's emotional journeys. I continued to care about Marcus, Dori, Darrel, and others but let go of what was not mine to carry. I shook off others' emotional clouds and stepped back onto my path.

Lingering wisps of sorrow still made an occasional presence, but simple delights were vibrant again. The flicker of candles and the scent of sugar cookies set the scene for wrapping gifts with red and green paper.

Soothing music played as I wrote hopeful messages on glittery cards. I was able to be more fully present for everyone in my life, including myself.

Caregivers don't have to give up their journey while holding hands with others during difficult times. We can promote our well-being and find balance even when life feels heavy. Effective caregiving includes space to nourish the hope and energy needed to thrive amid challenges. Healthy boundaries make this possible.

THE STRATEGY

UNDERSTAND HEALTHY BOUNDARIES

Boundaries clarify what we're responsible for. A wonderful example occurred when my sons, Joshua and Caleb, were young. Colorful Legos and Matchbox cars littered their bedroom floor. The stale odor of dirty clothes hit me as I entered to talk with them. I slipped on a rubber ball, caught myself, and hollered, "You need to clean your room now!"

The boys started yelling at each other as I left the room. I anticipated their argument would end with a fight and tears, but I was surprised by the silence. I crept back and peeked around the door frame to ensure they were okay. Their ingenuity stunned me. The boys used masking tape to draw a line down the middle of the room.

Joshua and Caleb established a boundary clarifying what each was responsible for. My mouth dropped as I saw them happily cleaning the room. We cannot always use tape, but we do need to know what we are and are not responsible for.

Boundaries relate to all aspects of life. They include physical, cognitive, and emotional limits that promote well-being. Taking time to walk, saving money for a trip, or saying "no" to a request all reveal a limit. So does refusing to be alone with someone who has violated our trust. Boundaries honor individuality and allow us to connect with others healthily and sustainably.

Consider the importance of boundaries during my Christmas week. Many responsibilities and limited time and energy increased the need for boundaries. Talking with Marcus was important, but I could've done a better job setting limits. I could've been more attentive and less concerned about what wasn't getting done if I mentally set a time limit and kindly explained it. A simple limit would've positively changed relationship dynamics.

Promoting boundaries isn't selfish because it increases positive connections. However, many individuals and organizations have insatiable needs and challenge healthy boundaries. A lack of understanding does not negate the need for limits. When we see boundaries as a negative, we risk taking on more than what is possible, including other people's emotional journeys.

What are we emotionally responsible for? As I provided end-of-life care for Dori, dealt with Darrel's complaints, and supported Marcus, was I responsible for assuming their emotions? We often equate caring with experiencing the same emotions as others, which is exhausting. Healthy boundaries honor the fact that we each have our emotional journeys and help us understand what we're responsible for.

Emotional boundaries are important whether we're taking care of loved ones or acquaintances. I know setting limits is hard with people we're especially close to. We more quickly lose perspective when our child is sobbing, our husband is stressed, or our parents are ill. However, we cannot effectively help others when we lose emotional distinctiveness. We risk becoming more focused on our own needs rather than those we're helping when we take on their emotional journeys.

Clarification between empathy and compassion can help us understand what we're emotionally responsible for. Empathy, in its original Greek, means to feel what others feel. It helps us connect with others, but we must keep empathy in perspective. Otherwise, we give up too much of ourselves.

Empathy fosters compassion, awareness of suffering, and a desire to end suffering. This honors emotional boundaries. We each are responsible for our own emotions and should allow others to experience and take responsibility for theirs. We can care about others, try to alleviate suffering, and experience our emotional journeys.

Promoting healthy boundaries, especially emotional ones, is easier to discuss than to do. Awareness is an important step towards honoring healthy boundaries and caring in sustainable ways. You can foster balance and resilience while helping others with some practical strategies to discern and set limits.

LIST BOUNDARY BENEFITS

A great starting point is to look at how healthy boundaries will help you and the people you're assisting. Write a list of the benefits so you can see that promoting limits is advantageous for everyone involved. A list may include:

- Our relationships will be more sustainable and enjoyable.
- I'll be able to take care of myself.
- I'm more likely to experience and share hope.
- We can know better who will do what.
- We'll better remember our responsibilities.
- We'll find our time together more meaningful.
- I'll have more energy to help and deal with challenges.
- I can be more authentic.
- I can allow others to be more authentic and express how they're feeling without it bothering me as much.
- I can say "no" when I don't feel right about something.
- Others will be more likely to honor my boundaries if I honor theirs.

You can use items from your list to explain how a boundary promotes everyone's well-being. Change is difficult, so be prepared for questions and opposition. Awareness of the positives will provide courage and inspiration when someone challenges efforts to establish boundaries.

CLARIFY RESPONSIBILITIES

We often sense we need to do something different to promote sustainability, but the "what" can be murky. We may feel tired often, get crabby more easily, or lose a sense of hope. We know this is not how we want to live, but we don't understand how to change. Clarifying our responsibilities helps us identify what boundaries can assist and how to implement them.

Creatively clarify responsibilities by using a yard or garden metaphor. On a piece of paper, draw a large square in the middle surrounded by other squares. The center square is your yard or garden and represents what you're responsible for. Neighboring squares identify other people's yards and responsibilities.

Consider what you're responsible for. This includes your roles' physical, cognitive, emotional, and social dynamics. Personal well-being should be at the top of your list. Our emotions also rank high. Remember, self-care is not selfish. Healthy caregivers provide better care. A complete list of responsibilities includes what we're obligated to provide for ourselves.

Write your responsibilities inside the center square. Have fun and decorate it with joyful flowers or wise trees. Include pesky weeds that you do not desire but must take care of. Use colors and shapes to personalize your yard. Make sure the space shows what you are responsible for.

After clarifying your responsibilities, identify other people's responsibilities. Designate surrounding yards for those you regularly interact with. This may include people you care for, family members, friends, coworkers, or colleagues. Write some responsibilities in their squares, such as attitude, health, and emotions. We recognize people's individuality and ability to be responsible by honoring their obligations.

What responsibilities in other people's yards do you tend to take on? Or what obligations in your yard do other people take on? It is too easy to assume other people's responsibilities when in a helping mode. Despite good intentions, spending too much time in other people's yards promotes unsustainable relationships. We unintentionally communicate, "You can't handle this," when repeatedly assuming other people's responsibilities.

Determine practical ways to take care of your responsibilities while helping others without taking on their duties. Consider what life looks like when you're thriving. Include values and purpose to reflect what is important. Write down some limits to help you spend more time in your yard and thrive as a caregiver.

Remember, your efforts aren't selfish and will benefit everyone involved. Be patient and persistent. It may seem easier to leap into other people's yards, especially when anxiety is involved. The following strategy can help you maintain calm by promoting emotional differentiation amid other people's anxiety and emotions.

MAINTAIN EMOTIONAL INDIVIDUALITY

Emotional differentiation helps us experience our journey while caring for others. We can remain calm and allow others to express their feelings when distinguishing between our emotions and those of others. A simple strategy to promote this involves picturing an energy field around each person.

Imagine a bubble around individuals whose emotions affect you. Envision your bubble and remember who you are. Think of a message you can use to promote emotional differentiation, such as "I am (name), I care, and I can feel differently." Imagine the emotional bubbles and remember your message when feeling anxious during an encounter. Those we help will still affect us, but we can influence how.

The conversation with Marcus weighed on me until I remembered what I was responsible for and permitted myself to be emotionally separate. I was able to provide ongoing care and support because of healthy boundaries. I experienced the simple joys and was fully present for other important relationships by honoring my responsibilities.

Understanding and promoting healthy boundaries takes time but is well worth the effort. When we care deeply about people, taking on their responsibilities and neglecting our own is easy. This often leads to burnout and compassion fatigue. We learn the hard way that caring about others doesn't take away the responsibility to care for ourselves. Sustainable, resilient caregiving requires healthy caregivers.

Your health is as important as that of anyone you help. We caregivers bring a wonderful gift to the world. We hold hands with people at the end of life, share encouraging words with those who have lost hope, and continue caring amid conflict. We honor who we are as individuals and the importance of connections with others by fostering healthy boundaries. As we promote our best, balanced self, we model the power of healthy caring to future caregivers.

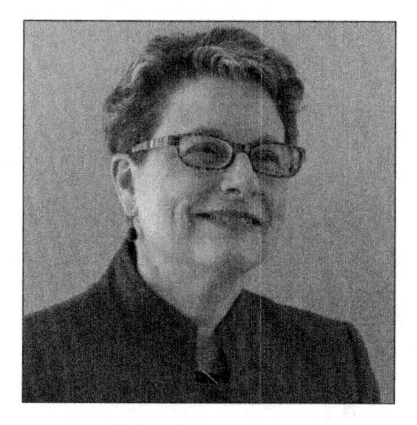

Karen Schuder, EdD, MDiv, MAM, has extensive experience promoting resilience and role sustainability through public speaking and coaching. Years of helping people during traumatic times, leading organizations, and working globally inform her work with people in personal and professional helping roles.

Karen offers life-changing concepts and practical strategies with an enjoyable, interactive approach. Her book, based on proven theories and research, provides a valuable resource for helping caregivers promote life balance and resilience.

This chapter includes information and excerpts from Karen's book *Resilient and Sustainable Caring: Your Guide to Thrive While Helping Others*, published by Whole Person Associates. You can purchase it through Amazon and other online providers.

Learn more about Karen's services and how to foster a purpose-driven culture characterized by resilience, positivity, and decreased anxiety at https://www.karenschuder.com

CHAPTER 6

Caregiver Burnout

WHAT IT IS AND HOW TO AVOID IT

Debbie DeMoss Compton, CCC, CCA

MY STORY

When did I get so tired? When was the last time I slept through the night? Do I even remember what it felt like to be rested? At this point, just soaking in a hot tub for 15 minutes would feel like a mini vacation! I have to find some help. There has to be a better way!

Earlier that day, I took Mom and my mother-in-law, Jean, to the doctor for their checkups. They're best friends and enjoy spending time together. I scheduled them both with the same physician to save time, trips, and confusion since I was a caregiver to both. Mom was living with vascular dementia, and Jean had Alzheimer's. Neither enjoyed going to the doctor; getting them to go was a battle.

Being a caregiver for two precious little ladies, both fighting different forms of dementia, is exhausting regardless of how much you love them or what plans you make.

I leave Mom (pants on and buttoning up her dress shirt) to check on Jean, who has decided to make a wardrobe change. I can see she's added a dress shirt with a button-up pajama shirt on top of it. To make things even more interesting, the right side of the pajama shirt is buttoned to the left side of the dress shirt!

"Let me help you with those buttons," I say while pretending all is normal. After some untangling, unbuttoning, removing, and re-buttoning, we're all set. As we enter the living room, Mom greets us in her pajamas!

"What happened to your clothes?" blurts out before I can stop my surprise. Mom's bewildered look causes me to instantly remember: *she has no idea.* I left her pajamas in the room, so she assumed it was time to put them on.

Note to self: take dirty clothes out of the room to avoid confusion.

Keeping them both in the same room, I managed to get both dressed, complete with glasses, hearing aids, teeth, and shoes. Off we go!

Both ladies get nervous at the thought of a doctor's visit. Nervousness can cause constant repetition, wringing hands, and outright rebellion. That day, I came up with a new approach.

Leaning close to Mom, I said, "The Doctor's visit is for Jean, but she gets anxious, so let's pretend it's for you." The cute smile and head nod reassured me Mom was on board.

As I helped Jean put her coat on, I whispered, "Mom gets so worried about going to the doctor. Can we pretend the visit is for you?" "Of course!" came the delighted response.

We all hold hands as we enter the garage, and I quickly place the stool down for my first passenger. My SUV can be challenging for short ladies with limited mobility, but the sturdy, fold-up stool solves the problem.

After both are loaded, buckled, and with water bottles in their respective doors, I finally climb in. I utilize the door cup holders, as drinks placed in the center console are too confusing. I don't enjoy explaining which drink is whose 500 times (another lesson learned the hard way).

Both screens in the headrests come on and the ladies are happily watching Doris Day and Rock Hudson.

Mom comments repeatedly on how pretty Doris Day's hats and dresses are. Jean smiles and agrees with her friend, never getting irritated at the constant repetition.

I need to be more like her; she's so patient with Mom. Sigh.

We disembark in reverse order. Once one lady is safely out, we hold hands while walking to the other side of the SUV. Then she holds the door for me (so she won't wander off) while I get the second one out.

Holding hands, we march, dance, or stroll, depending on the mood, into the doctor's office. Distractions are everywhere: a flower, a bird, a strange crack in the concrete, a nice car, a cute baby, and seemingly a million other things. Every distraction causes our feet to stop walking, and we stop to comment on whatever it may be.

Each restart of movement takes encouragement and a gentle tug on their hands.

It's not that far! Can we please just walk?

We finally get checked in and stop six times to look at distractions before, at last, arriving in the waiting room next door. We're in the early stages of our journey, yet I can feel my tension building.

They can't help it. Stay calm. Breathe.

After returning magazines to the rack, gathering purses, and holding hands, we marched to the examination room.

Once the doctor arrives, each lady tells him it's the other one's appointment. I smile innocently, and he laughs as he gives me a thumbs-up sign.

"Since you're already here, why don't I go ahead and give you a quick check, too?" the Dr. tells each lady. They reluctantly agree so as not to appear rude.

Now, I can take a deep breath and relax in the hard plastic chair for a moment. The doctor can examine them. *Mission accomplished.*

After going through many days like that and nights of continually interrupted sleep, it takes a toll on the body. I didn't know the term at the time, but I was experiencing caregiver burnout. See if you can relate.

Caregiver burnout is defined as a state of complete mental, physical, and emotional exhaustion.

It creeps up on you like a frog placed in a pan of cool water. Everything is going okay. The water is nice; the caregiving job is not that hard.

Days roll by, and your freedom diminishes due to increased caregiving responsibilities. It's not easy, but you can handle it. Then, the heat gets turned up a little. Your loved one gets worse. Things previously done with ease now seem impossible. Friends become scarce and "me time" disappears, and the heat or stress rises.

More issues come up. You may get irritated, but you hold it in, or you may explode. Going anywhere takes so much longer than it used to. There are so many things to remember now, and the temperature rises yet again.

If I can get some sleep or a little help, I'll be okay, you reason. But the help doesn't come, and the sleep is constantly interrupted. And the water starts to boil.

You snap at your loved one, kick the dog, get angry because your head hurts and your back aches, and there's no end in sight. Then you feel guilty because you lost your temper. Guilty because you don't have enough patience. Guilty because you hurt their feelings—just guilty.

I'm not sure I can make it! I'm not strong enough. I need to do better.

You've experienced unrelieved stress for an extended period of time, and now, my friend, you're in full-blown caregiver burnout.

Exhaustion sets in. Even if you have a chance to sleep, you can't turn your brain off to actually sleep. Stress causes muscles to tense up, and it's hard to get them to relax again. Headaches and digestive issues can become regular occurrences. You may have high blood pressure, difficulty concentrating, or become irritated at even small things.

Body aches and cramping can occur for no apparent reason other than the stress you're enduring. You need to find relief—fast.

It's important to recognize that you need help. Caregiving is **not** a solo adventure.

Raising a child takes a village, and so does caring for a loved one.

THE STRATEGY

May I offer some suggestions? You may not like all of them, and that's okay. Try the ones that feel good to you, but please try several. You may be surprised at the benefits you experience!

JOURNALING

Give journaling a try. Write down a funny thing or two that happened or was said. Write out your feelings. Be honest with yourself and release your worries, anger, depression, or whatever you're feeling to the page.

Journaling has been scientifically proven to lower stress, offer clearer focus, increase our ability to develop a workable solution, and be a great brain dump, freeing our brains of all negativity.

"Journaling is a tool to put our experiences, thoughts, beliefs, and desires into language, and in doing so, it helps us understand and grow and make sense of them," says Joshua Smyth, a distinguished professor of bio-behavioral health and medicine at Penn State University.

MINDSET

There is plenty to be angry or negative about every day. Depressing thoughts surround us. Why not choose to focus on the positive? The funny or sweet stuff is there; sometimes, we have to look a little harder to find it.

Here's an example: Mom was having a rough morning. She didn't want to go to the optometrist and couldn't care less that her glasses weren't strong enough anymore. She wanted to sleep in, so she resisted me at every turn.

By some miracle, we arrived on time. As we sat down after checking in, tired from the struggle and leaning forward in my chair, I couldn't believe what I saw. Mom had one brown and one black shoe on!

How did that happen?! My inner critic screamed.

In this instance, I quickly subdued the critic and mentally pointed out the facts. *We made it here on time. Mom is fully dressed, with her glasses and dentures. So what if her shoes don't match? No one will notice. And if they do, I'll say, "She has another pair just like them at home!" This is a win!*

Recognize it may not be funny at the time, but it will be in the future. I believe the key to happiness is to laugh sooner.

If you want to improve your mood, make a habit of writing down at least three things you're thankful for each day. Don't allow yourself to repeat anything that week, and you'll experience a more significant mood lift. It changes your focus, which changes your outlook.

Your mindset plays a vital role in caregiving. As Henry Ford famously said, "Whether you think you can or you think you can't, you're right."

Determine to have a good day regardless of what happens. I know it isn't easy. I know you're tired, but I believe you're stronger than you know.

FAITH

My dad pastored small country churches. I grew up in church. We went Sunday morning, Sunday night, Wednesday night, every night of revival, and every morning of vacation Bible school. I've held every position in the church except pastor and deacon. I asked Jesus to come into my heart at the age of eight, and I've never regretted it.

What does that have to do with caregiving? Everything.

I was scrubbing the bathroom floor for the third time that day, tears streaming down my face. My body ached from lifting and transferring her body, which no longer functioned correctly. I was beyond tired, unsure I could go another step. I couldn't see an end in sight or the relief I so desperately needed.

It's in those moments of deep sadness and exhaustion that God's word lifts me up, gives me strength for the day, and encourages me to go on. Scriptures memorized years earlier come back to mind when I need them most.

"Greater is He that is in me than he that is in the world." 1 John 4:4

"His mercies are new every morning, great is your faithfulness." Lamentations 3:22-23

"I can do ALL things," *even scrub this bathroom floor for the third time,* "through Christ who gives me strength." Philippians 4:13

With a renewed knowledge that God is in control and that He will supply my every need, I rise to face the next challenge. If you want to know more about that, please reach out. I would be delighted to share with you!

SUPPORT GROUPS OR PRIVATE DISCUSSIONS

Support groups can be a big help as you share experiences with others in similar situations. You can learn from each other, empathize, and maybe even offer a workable solution. Support groups are offered both online and in person. Google the diagnosis plus (+) "support groups near me" to find local gatherings.

I deliver one-on-one Zoom consultations to offer ideas, encouragement, and laughter. Your first session is free so we can get acquainted and you can get a feel for how it works. My clients love it because they can call while their loved one sleeps or watches TV. There's no dressing up, no travel time, and no hassle. Sometimes, they need to talk to someone who understands; sometimes, it's to gain insight, and other times, they need to know where to find help or resources. Whatever the need, I'm trained and experienced and have lived your journey.

BREATHWORK

Another tip I'll offer today is breathing. It may sound silly, but I—and many of my clients—have witnessed its benefits. When you're stressed, angry, irritated, or just in a foul mood, this technique will help. It lowers your heart rate, increases the oxygen in your brain so you can think more clearly, and helps you be more creative. You don't need anyone to help you do it, and you can do it anywhere. Plus, it's simple!

Ready to try it? After you've read through the steps, you'll practice it with your eyes closed. You can also do it with them open, but in my experience, it takes longer and is more challenging to achieve the calm state you desire. There are too many distractions with your eyes open, and your focus is not as concentrated.

Breathe slowly in for four counts through your nose. Hold that breath for a slow four count, and then exhale through the mouth for a slow four count. Repeat at least three times.

As you breathe in, imagine you are breathing in pure, clean, calming air. Hold it to let it seep into your brain, filling the brain with fresh oxygen. Then, exhale stress, anger, or any negative emotions that are present.

The more you practice four-part breathing, the better you will become at it, and the faster you can move to a more relaxed state. Remember to focus on your breathing and your thoughts. Shut out distractions as much as possible and focus on slow, steady breathing in clean, calming air. Hold that air for a slow four-count before exhaling all the toxins out through your mouth.

Many other relaxation techniques will benefit you as a caregiver or a person in the workforce today. Or even as a human living in these stressful times! More are on my website: https://thePurpleVine.com/reduce-stress/

COLORING BOOKS

Adult coloring books are a great activity you can do with your loved one or individually. I created several and let my granddaughters enjoy coloring with my mom, who was in the late stages of vascular dementia. Coloring was an activity they could all do together and enjoy. It helped Mom with hand-eye coordination, decision-making, creativity, distraction, relaxation, socialization, and the joy of seeing her masterpiece completed.

For the caregiver, coloring can also bring calmness, as the mind focuses on creating and forgets the stresses of the day.

Tami, a long-time friend of mine, uses my *Faith Lives Here* coloring book to help pass the time while undergoing chemo treatments. She appreciates the distraction and also the creation of something beautiful and unique. Give it a try; you might be surprised.

OTHER SERVICES

Contact your local DHS (Google "DHS+" your state) Area Centers for Aging, Adult Day Care Programs, Senior Living Facilities, or other services to find out what is available. There are Meals on Wheels, transportation services, and many FREE things!

If research feels daunting, ask your physician what services are available in your area. You can also book a complimentary first Zoom call with me, and I'll look it up for you. The point is that you have options, and support and programs are available in most areas.

Any steps you take toward better self-care are good.

When you are exhausted, you aren't the best caregiver. To show up and provide quality care, we must first care for ourselves. I know it seems impossible at times; I've been there, but the good news is, I've learned to do better, and so can you.

I created ways to make life safer and easier, and I gladly share them with my clients. You are doing a wonderful thing in caring for your loved one. It is not easy, but it can be easier. Reach out and I would be honored to help you.

Thank you for reading! I pray strength, compassion, and peace fill your days!

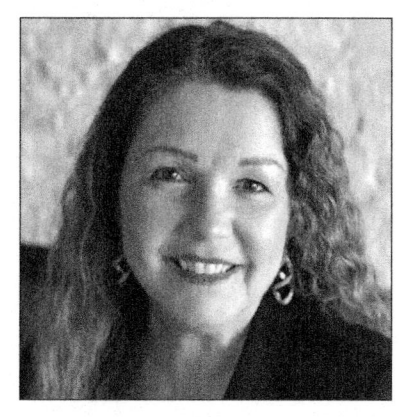

Debbie Compton is a three-time primary caregiver for parents with different forms of dementia. She cared for her Dad with Parkinson's until he passed in his home and her mother-in-law with Alzheimer's until she passed in Debbie and her husband's home. Debbie's Mom, who was the first to get dementia, was also the last of the three to go to heaven, leaving this past September. Her sweet Mom battled vascular dementia for 21 years!

Debbie speaks on caregiver and dementia issues from first-hand experience and professional training. She brings encouragement, hope, and laughter to an often stressful caregiver journey.

Mrs. Compton has been a Community Educator for the Alzheimer's Association since 2017. She is also a Certified Caregiver Consultant and Advocate. She founded The Purple Vine, which aims to empower caregivers to reduce stress, block burnout, and learn to laugh again.

Besides playing with her grandbabies, Debbie's favorite thing is educating others through Zoom chats. She will have you laughing as you learn. Bring your worries or concerns to the private coaching call and leave feeling encouraged and refreshed.

She's authored nine books previous to this one. Most are for caregiver support, and all are due to a family member in need. Whether you need an Activity book for a child, a lovable llama journal for your teen, or an Adult coloring book, she's got you covered. There's also a thick journal created for caregivers to ease their stress and recover joy.

In her book "Caregiving: How to Hold On While Letting Go," Debbie shares her hard-earned knowledge, inventions, and faith. She helps readers find blessings and humor still present in their lives by sharing much of hers. Visit Debbie's website and blog at https://www.thePurpleVine.com

Contact Debbie at Deb@ThePurpleVine.com

Connect on LinkedIn at https://linkedin.com/in/DebbieDCompton

Instagram https://www.instagram.com/Debbie_Compton1

FaceBook https://www.facebook.com/Caregiving.Book

Pinterest http://www.pinterest.com/compton1788

CHAPTER 7

Safety First

WHEN IS IT TIME TO STOP DRIVING?

Kathleen Plummer Gordon, MSW

MY STORY

Everything was fine with my dad's driving until he shocked us. My father backed up from his reserved parking spot and crashed into a parked car. When he realized what he had done, he quickly shifted the car into drive and gunned it back toward his parking spot. He kept moving over the curb, up an embankment, and into an apartment building. He was then able to reverse the car and stop at the parking spot where he started from.

As a social worker, I've counseled many families grappling with care for their elderly loved ones and concerns about their loved ones driving. The anguish hit me on a personal level in the summer of 2015. My mother fell ill, and for three months, my family was faced with making decisions about health care as we watched her slow physical decline. The eight of us children were concerned about how our dad was coping with the love of his life slowly leaving this world. Little signs of his mild cognitive impairment (MCI) were creeping up on us, like when my dad would say, "Where did I put my keys?" or "Where did I put my wallet?" several times a day.

Our 91-year-old father, who had a shuffling, unsteady gait, was telling us he was fine driving. We watched him as he held onto the furniture or a wall to maneuver around my parents' apartment. My dad only agreed to get a handicap placard for his car because, as he stated, "It would be convenient for your mother." He didn't think it would be right for him to take up a space for a handicapped person if he was capable of walking.

My father was not the type to ask for help. By this time, he already had a couple of falls and scraped up his head and knees. Once he fell walking home from the grocery store and a kind gentleman drove him home and walked him to his front door. He was encouraged to use a walker but thought he was fine without one. *So stubborn!* All of us were concerned about him driving. One of my brothers passed him once in traffic, noticing my dad was driving slowly in the right-hand lane and holding up traffic. The four of us who lived in town (Margaret, Susan, Will, and I) offered to drive him to make things easier. The other four siblings out of town (Don, Charlie, Alice, and Judy) each visited twice that summer. He gladly accepted a ride but always checked to make sure he wasn't putting us out of our way.

We talked to him about a plan where one of us drove him to see my mother every day at the rehab center or the hospital, then took him to lunch and drove him home. Another sibling picked him up later in the day to take him out for dinner or bring food to him. He agreed with our plan, and I think he appreciated our company. He always thanked us for driving him and said, "You kids are doing too much."

We took turns driving our dad wherever he needed to go for the next two months. It was time-consuming and exhausting for all of us to coordinate care for our parents; so many phone calls and text messages between the eight of us! It seemed like everything else in life was on hold. We've told each other many times how glad we are to have a large number of siblings to depend on. We thought we were covered because he wasn't going anywhere anyway, or so we thought.

My younger brother, Will, had a couple of conversations with our dad about when the time might be to retire from driving. Daddy assured Will that he'd let him know when he was not comfortable driving. He would say, "I'm not quite there yet."

My two older brothers, Don and Charlie, talked with him about having someone else take over the driving. That didn't go over very well. When one offered to drive him in his car, he became angry and accused them of trying to take his car keys from him. They were concerned enough to fill out a medical form and report him to the DMV to have his driver's license revoked. However, my father's physician was unwilling to sign the form. The plan to fill out an "unsafe driver report" was discussed and was on hold at this point.

One day, it was my turn to drive Daddy to see Mom at the rehab center. When I dropped him off that afternoon back at his apartment, I reminded him that Margaret, my sister, would be coming by later with dinner. That evening, I got a call from my younger sister, Susan, explaining the horrifying vehicle accident Daddy was in without even getting out of the parking lot. I braced myself for the terrible news.

We are talking about our dad, who taught all eight of us to drive and never caused a vehicle accident.

Miraculously, no one was injured. When the police officer came to take the report, my father could tell him the date. He could name the current president and was polite and cooperative. This little bit of information was enough for the police officer to conclude that my dad was alert and oriented enough to drive.

Are you kidding me?

There was no mention of taking his license or suggesting he not drive. I'm sure my father's anxiety about my mother was all-consuming to the point where it interfered with his ability to complete daily tasks competently.

I was at my dad's apartment the day the insurance adjuster came. Also, there was the young lady whose car my father damaged. She came over, hugged me, and said, "I hope your dad is okay." I let her know he was fine. And then I tearfully apologized on behalf of my father. She wasn't worried in the least about her car. My dad's car had significant damage in the front and rear. It was totaled. I saw the cracks in the apartment building, signs of where the front of his car smashed in.

How could someone with a perfect driving record cause this much damage?

The insurance agent looked at me hesitantly and asked if my father would be driving again. I assured him, "Absolutely not!" The insurance agent pried open the car trunk with a crowbar. I collected the few belongings my father kept there: a toolbox, a pair of shoes, and a couple of rags, and carried them to his apartment. Daddy looked confused and asked me where I got the items. When I told him they were from the trunk of his car, he stated he was certain these items did not belong to him. He even told me he had never seen the toolbox.

Another sign of his cognitive decline.

The insurance adjuster brought papers for my father to sign, explaining in his professional manner that the insurance company would file two separate claims: one to cover the cost of the damage to the other vehicle and the second for the damage to the building. As the insurance agent and I waited silently, my father read through all the report details. He signed on the bottom line without any questions. We informed him that his car was being sold, and the insurance agent gave him a check. He was confused again, saying, "I'm the one who caused the accident. I don't deserve any money."

Several times after this incident, my father told us, "Maybe I should just get another car." Fortunately, he didn't. The double accident was the last time my father got behind the wheel of a vehicle.

We had a plan and took steps to prevent him from driving, except taking the keys. When I talked with my dad later about where he planned to drive, he said, "I was just going down the street to get a hamburger." When I reminded him that Margaret was on the schedule to bring dinner, he said he had forgotten. Maybe he just wanted to drive after not having the experience for two months. It didn't matter; he had poor decision-making and was out of the driving practice. He shouldn't have been behind the wheel.

Post-accident, I remember several occasions while driving my dad he would comment, "Oh I've never seen this street before." I gently pointed out one or two businesses and then told him the name of the street we were approaching at the next traffic light. He usually responded with, "Oh yeah, now I remember."

More cognitive decline.

After experiencing this terrifying situation with my own family, I decided to take the opportunity to help other families prevent this exact scenario from happening to them.

Many people look forward to the day when they can retire from work and live leisurely. Regarding retirement from driving, some people can plan and hand over the keys, while others (like my father) struggle with losing independence and control. Families caring for an elderly loved one may be struggling to balance independence with caregiving. Being in a caregiver role puts the adult child in the position of making some decisions about instrumental activities of daily living, many times referred to as IADLs. One of the IADLs that is difficult for many seniors to hand over is driving. After all, driving is a significant form of independence, and who wants to give that up? Telling Mom or Dad they need to stop driving is not the conversation we look forward to with our elderly parents. Balancing safety and independence for seniors can be challenging. Regarding driving retirement, here are some tips to help adult children make these decisions.

While working as a Senior Living Consultant, I occasionally got calls from someone out of town who just returned from a visit with their parents (usually during the holidays). The adult child would speak in a panic mode about how their mother or father has declined so much since their last visit (six months or a year ago). They were in shock because "She always told me everything was fine when we spoke on the phone, but now that I've seen her, I know she should not drive." Then, there was a request for help finding a senior living community quickly, and that's why it's so important to have some local eyes on our elderly loved ones.

I had a lady call me concerned about her father driving. He'd often drive to a place he had been to and get lost (not on purpose). He'd then call his wife and ask for directions without being able to explain his location. He didn't have GPS in his car. Quite scary!

A friend told me about her family trying to get her father to stop driving. He refused, so they did things to manipulate the car, like disconnecting battery cables or hiding his keys. He was a mechanic, so he knew how to fix his car. She said they deactivated the electric garage door from opening, and that worked for a while. Eventually, he figured it out. When he learned about a woman who needed a car, he gladly donated it to her. Problem solved!

One client told me she was concerned about her husband's temper. I said, "Please tell me he's not driving." She tried to assure me he was fine. "He just had one little incident the week before when he backed into the garage door." I shared my family's story and encouraged her to take his car keys. She was afraid to because she didn't want him to be angry with her. In this case, her daughter stepped in and talked with her father. It was tough, but she stood her ground and told her father that everyone's safety had to be a top priority. She was able to get the keys.

There are numerous stories, and they go on and on. The common factor here is a decline in driving competence with senior drivers. I've heard many clients say they don't want their parents to be angry with them. When we are in the midst of emotional, gut-wrenching issues that suck up our time and energy, it's easier to go along with the sweet, frail, elderly person who tries to convince us they'll be fine instead of taking the time to make sure the car keys are not available. Driving is not an option for them. Talk with your loved one about other options for transportation.

THE STRATEGY

Sometimes, seniors are worried that if they stop driving, they'll lose out on social events. They may feel they're a burden to their family members, or they may feel a loss of control and spontaneity without a car. Many senior communities provide transportation for the residents to medical appointments, grocery stores, and social outings. Many of these senior communities offer a boatload of social activities as well. Check the resource page.

Medications can negatively impact a person's driving. For example, many medicines used to treat chronic pain have a side effect of confusion and memory issues. If you know your loved one is taking medication, it may be helpful to have a comprehensive medication evaluation with their healthcare provider. Some seniors will be confident driving in their familiar area, getting to the grocery store or church. Driving on the freeway could be overwhelming for them. Some seniors with a diagnosis of early-stage Alzheimer's or another form of dementia may still be able to handle driving. However, when the disease progresses and affects memory and decision-making skills, it's time for driving retirement. A newer vehicle with a backup camera can make parking and backing up easier. Avoiding rush hour traffic or highly congested areas may help senior drivers.

Rather than engaging in ongoing arguments, seniors and their adult children can start conversations about transportation needs. Planning and action can prevent tragic situations like my father's. This is a huge public safety issue. No one benefits from an older, confused driver with slower processing and reaction times.

Signs and symptoms to look for:
- The car has a few dents and scratches.
- The senior is very anxious while driving.
- The senior is constantly riding the brake.
- Other drivers are often honking at the senior driver.
- The senior is nervous about backing up.
- The senior drives way under or way over the speed limit.

In many cities, Area Councils on Aging provide transportation for seniors for medical appointments and grocery shopping. There is no cost for the service.

Some Veterans Hospitals provide a driving evaluation called Capacity and Fitness to Drive a Motor Vehicle at no cost to the veteran. A driving evaluation in the community may cost $500.00 to $600.00 (not usually covered by insurance).

If you feel your loved one is driving unsafely but refuses to turn over the keys, you can file an "Unsafe Driver" report with your state's DMV. This is different than a medical report. Do not worry about hurting their feelings or how angry they'll be with you. This situation is undoubtedly challenging, but there are no second chances. Placing safety as the top priority is the best decision for everyone. When your gut tells you something is not good, pay attention and act!

Self-driving vehicles are still in the infancy stage. It's not recommended for an elderly, frail person to try this on their own. A ride-sharing app such as Uber or Lyft may be beneficial. For those who need a van, nonemergency medical transport is an option.

In some states, drivers 65 and older must renew their licenses every five years and take a vision test. Every state is different, so check with your state transportation department regarding the rules for senior drivers. Handicap placards can be helpful for seniors who need assistance getting in and out of a vehicle, have a severe heart condition, or are on oxygen.

Safe senior driving helps everyone.

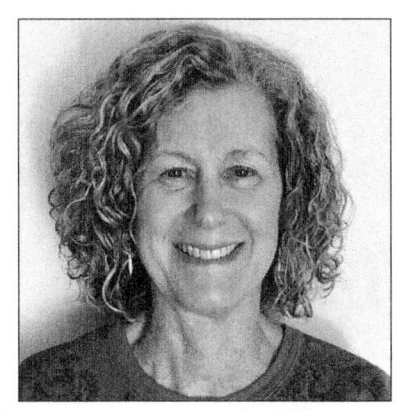

Kathleen Plummer Gordon, MSW, is a retired licensed clinical social worker and a senior advocate. She has provided community presentations on Senior Care and end-of-life issues and counseled families grappling with elder care issues such as locating senior living communities, driving, home services, and family relationships. Kathleen has experience in Medical Foster Home for Veterans, investigating guardianship and conservatorship court cases, school social work, and psychotherapy private practice. Kathleen is available to give presentations on senior issues.

Contact Kathleen at

Wildkataz81@gmail.com

https://www.linkedin.com/in/kathleen-gordon-153a06223

CHAPTER 8

The Art of Financial Self-Defense

STRATEGIES TO PROTECT THE ELDERLY FROM EXPLOITATION

Michael Lewis, CFA MBA

MY STORY

Stress. It impacts financial decision-making and can destroy a family's legacy.

With financial responsibility comes great temptation and easy access. Even good people can do bad things, particularly under duress. No one is immune to being misled, even victimized, by people we like, admire, or even trust.

Whenever I went to San Francisco, I always stopped in on Raymond, the firm's leading producer on the West Coast. All his clients loved him. Senior management loved his bottom-line contribution. *Everybody loves Raymond.*

I knew Raymond was great with people. I also knew he was not good with numbers. Ray often asked me to help reconcile his accounts. When the regional VP resigned, the company decided to promote Raymond. It made sense. Ray has a track record of success and is already located in SF.

What could possibly go wrong?

Robert, the CEO, asked me what I thought of promoting Ray. I expressed my concern. "Ray is a great salesperson, but I fear he'll not make a great executive. If we promote him without proper training and support, we may be setting him up for failure."

"You worry too much. Ray has always come through for us. He is very resourceful."

The first time I saw Ray after his promotion, he looked different. He wasn't the normally sartorial, splendidly dressed man to whom I was accustomed. *You need a haircut.*

"I miss sales," Ray lamented. "Now all I do is go to meetings and prepare management reports I don't really understand."

"I'm concerned for you, Ray. I think you may be in over your head. Why don't you ask for help?"

"If I ask for help, I'll get fired. Don't worry Mike, I'll figure it out."

"How's the Mrs.?"

"We're getting a divorce. This is going to cost me big."

I returned to New York and reported back to the CEO. He also expressed concern for Raymond and asked me to keep an eye on the San Francisco office. "You know what to look for," he said as we reviewed the agenda for my next trip.

There were two aspects I had to monitor: Ray's change in behavior and his access to a debt budget, including some discretionary payment limits.

With Ray, the changes started off subtly. He used to get his haircut every week, but now he gets it every month. He always went out to lunch; now, he brought lunch from home. He used to wear a Rolex, now a Timex.

Makes sense, given his marital situation.

Then he started coming late to work. Soon, he began missing meetings. One day, I was sure he smelled of alcohol. I was running out of time.

An audit of Ray's corporate expense account confirmed my worst fears. His expenses for the past six months have been steadily increasing. He was paying his personal bills with company money.

I presented the evidence to senior management, and Ray was dismissed, but not before he could embezzle over $250,000 from the company.

Hindsight: Senior management put the wrong guy into a management position. A system of checks and balances revealed the irregularities and curtailed the damage.

THE STRATEGY

According to a CNN poll conducted in June 2023, 73% of Americans worry about money. Think that number has gone down since then?

Here is another fun fact: the number one reason for divorce is infidelity. The number two reason? Finances.

Imagine having to make a life-or-death decision with significant financial implications while in a highly agitated and emotional state. Maybe you don't have to imagine, as you are already reading this book. Welcome to the life of a financial caregiver. Read on for more insights into this critical role.

Worrying may lead to stress. Stress may lead to bad choices. Bad choices may lead to financial problems. Financial problems may lead to desperate measures.

In 2022, there were 88,262 complaints of fraud from people aged sixty or over, resulting in $3.1 billion in losses, according to the Federal Bureau of Investigation (FBI) Internet Crime Complaint Center. The most popular are:

- **Government impersonation scams.** Nothing can scare an elderly person more than the fear of government action. Scammers will use web addresses that appear legitimate. They will call and threaten legal action. Please be aware that the IRS will never call.

- **Computer support scams.** My mom loves to play Spider solitaire. She will often complain about viruses and popups. One of the popups looked like a virus detection warning and said, 'Click here to remove all viruses.' Fortunately, I witnessed this and prevented my mom from clicking the icon. Had she, her computer, and all the data would've been compromised.

- **Grandparent scam.** The unsuspecting victim receives a call from someone pretending to be their grandchild. Guess who, Grandma? When Grandma guesses, the caller uses the name to gain trust.
- **Sweepstakes and lottery scams.** Imposters call and claim that you have won the grand prize. All you have to do is provide your name, date of birth, address, and social security number so we can verify you before sending a check.
- **Robocall scams.** Often, callers begin by asking the caller to verify their name. They record the callers' 'Yes' and use it to make purchases.

Note that strangers are not the only scammers in the world of elder fraud. Trusted vendors, friends, and family members can resort to drastic measures when pushed to their extreme.

I remember watching my wife, Sharon, having a "Groundhog Day conversation" over and over with her dad. Finally, she threw up her hands and pleaded with me to help her. That night, Sharon realized that her dad's situation would only worsen. "If you don't help me with my dad, I will go insane and take you with me." (Sharon loves the movie Beetlejuice. Please read Chapter 15, *Stop the World I Want to Get Off*, for additional information on how to stay sane.)

It's important to take a moment to differentiate the role of a financial caregiver, as this person may or may not oversee the medical and emotional care of the loved one. The financial caregiver may also be or may not be a family member. In these situations, an independent fiduciary may be hired to help navigate the multiple considerations, decisions, and requirements.

Is proximity to a loved one the primary criteria for the role of financial caregiver? Not necessarily. Managing someone else's financial affairs relies more on skill and dedication than location.

As a family member or as hired expertise, here is a sampling of the responsibilities that a financial caregiver may assume, along with descriptions of the risks you run when these responsibilities are not managed correctly:

- **Review mail:** Financial loss can occur simply by ignoring or failing to take action. Scammers that impersonate the IRS sow fear and stress in the elderly, who often will pay on the spot rather than question the letter's validity. Credit card companies send offers that require no action to accept but can take months to dispute. Be suspicious, and look for clues on the validity of the information, deadlines, and why personal data is requested before responding.
- **File for government benefits:** If you're of social security age and assume the government will automatically enroll you, guess again. Timing is key if you want to maximize benefits and avoid penalties. If you are claiming a disability, there may be time constraints that must be met, or potential benefits may be lost.
- **Pay Premiums:** If a life insurance policy lapses because of a failure to make a payment, coverage will be denied if the claim occurs after the grace period. In the case of long-standing life insurance policies, they may be prohibitively expensive to replace.
- **Reconcile accounts:** Whether fraud or an honest mistake, the evidence will reveal itself in the financial records. Conducting a monthly reconciliation will ensure that errors are corrected, late fees are reversed, and questionable charges are properly researched.
- **Manage investments:** Significant and unnecessary tax consequences can be incurred if investments aren't appropriately liquidated. Monies may be subject to inappropriate market risk, and their ability to meet future cash needs may be jeopardized. Failure to properly take your required minimum distribution (RMD) may result in a penalty of 25% of the RMD if a retirement account is involved.
- **File tax returns:** The penalty for filing late is 5% of your tax liability for each month late, up to a maximum of 25%. Need I say more?
- **Disburse funds:** The financial caregiver may need access to their client's ATM, checkbook, credit cards, and online accounts.

Take this opportunity to consolidate banking relationships and safely dispose of unwanted credit cards. Eliminate unnecessary banking relationships and reduce service fees and opportunities for fraud.

"The great lesson in microeconomics is to discriminate between when technology is going to help you and when it's going to kill you." Charlie Munger.

Recently, we got my mother an Alexa. It's a great companion. Ask her to play music, tell you the weather, or tell a story. Alexa does it all.

Unfortunately, Alexa is always listening even if you are not aware.

"Grandma, your Pringles are stale. You need more," our eldest son complained.

"What flavor do you like?"

"Please order more plain Pringles."

Wouldn't you know it? In two days, Amazon delivered an order of plain Pringles. Good thing he didn't ask for a Maserati.

Technology can simplify the management of household finances, protect your loved ones from computer scammers, and allow your support team to share critical time-sensitive information and communicate with each other efficiently. Please read Chapter 2 on how to build your support team.

Here are some tips for upgrading and securing your family's technology:

1. Procure an app to facilitate the sharing of official records. Scan all necessary documents (will, trust agreements, insurance policies, annuity contracts, financial institution login/passwords, etc.) and provide access only to those who need it. Please read Chapter 4 for additional estate planning information.
2. Install and maintain virus protection software on all computers.
3. Set up automatic bill payment.
4. Turn off the online shopping capability on any personal devices in the home.
5. Use an app to manage and securely share passwords with others.
6. Apply all security patches and upgrades in a timely manner.
7. Assign someone the role of system administrator and provide them with remote access. If you cannot do it, hire a professional.

A good IT support person has been known to save a marriage or two.

"You can always trust a dishonest man to be dishonest. Honestly, it's the honest ones you have to watch out for." Captain Jack Sparrow.

We previously suggested that one need not be local to be someone's financial caregiver. That being said, if you are local and anyone in the family suspects a financial predator is running loose, then a strong local presence is required. The designated 'security guard' should get to know all regular visitors. Only by establishing a benchmark can you detect changes in behavior. Here are some suggestions:

- **Maintain a visitor's log.** Note the names, date, time, and length of stay.
- **Conduct a monthly inventory** (including prescription medications) of items in the house. Where did that Steuben glass figurine go? Is the client taking the medications, or is one of the children stealing them?
- **Never leave the client unaccompanied with guests.** All it takes is 'just log me into your account' or 'just sign this' and all funds and confidential data are at risk.
- **Look for changes.** Is someone visiting more than usual? Has someone experienced a radical change in appearance or personal grooming?
- **Report back regularly** to the other family members on the client's condition, a summary of visitors, and the results of the physical count.

A financial caregiver's mismanagement of any of the responsibilities described above, even unintentionally, can cause great harm to the loved one, their immediate family, and future generations. If you are overwhelmed or unsure, hire an independent fiduciary to help you navigate the multiple considerations, decisions, and requirements. In doing so, you can have increased confidence and peace of mind.

Protect your loved ones and their legacy. Connect with Michael Lewis, CFA MBA: https://inphone.co/michael-lewis

Want to learn how stress may be impacting your financial decision-making? This questionnaire will measure your attitude towards risk and reward, key drivers in any decision. Behavioral Finance Questionnaire: https://atlaspoint.qualtrics.com/jfe/form/SV_0JTZ13ZZ40rvZps/?uid=zsi3yo8OB

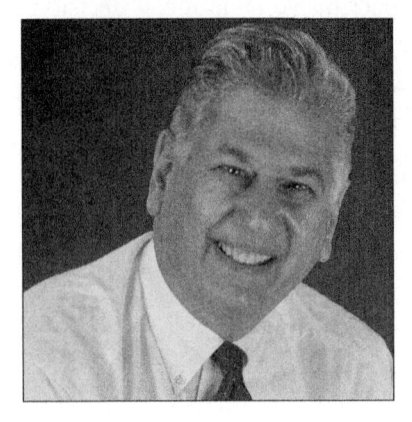

Over Michael's career, he learned how Wall Street works from the inside, assisting international banks such as BNY Mellon and institutional fund managers such as SEI Investments in managing risks and improving returns using technology.

Frustrated by the difference in service quality received by the wealthy vs. the 'rest of us,' Michael and his wife Sharon founded Tutor Financial Advisors, LLC., recently integrated with Family Legacy Financial Solutions, a family wealth office.

The name Tutor Financial Advisors reflects education's importance in financial planning. Tutor's mission is to assist families in cementing their legacy and transitioning wealth to future generations in a tax-efficient manner.

- Family Legacy believes that estate planning is for everyone, regardless of personal situation. They feel that we all have a responsibility to our children and grandchildren to pass on our values, virtues, and wisdom. At the same time, we must prepare them to assume the responsibility that comes with inheriting wealth.

- Each of us will be a caregiver at some point, making it critical to understand our choices and partner with those most qualified to assist us. As caregivers, we must also be able to recognize behaviors that indicate additional care requirements or cautionary messages regarding the financial security of our loved ones.

Michael sits on the boards of the East North Carolina Red Cross and the Jewish Federation of Raleigh-Cary. He educates patients at recovery centers on financial literacy and further advises families who are financially trying to balance the expenses incurred when a loved one is experiencing addictive behaviors.

Michael enjoys a good round of golf and BBQ when not working on his business. He is particularly fond of his Big Green Egg and the crust he achieves on his briskets.

Connect with Michael Lewis, CFA MBA

Website: https://inphone.co/michael-lewis

Email: Michael@familylegacync.com

CHAPTER 9

Hands-On Care

ESSENTIAL TIPS FOR BATHING AND EATING

Daneika D. Farmer

MY STORY

"No, you are not. You nigger," he replied.

Gulp. *I know he just didn't.*

I took a deep breath as my eyes filled with tears, then blinked several times to keep the tears from running down the sides of my face.

"I'm sorry, sir. I've been assigned to help you get out of bed and cleaned up for the day before your family gets here. I know you are probably ready to eat breakfast, too."

"You nigger, I told you, no you aren't," he replied again.

Father God, in the name of Jesus, please touch this man.

I took a deep breath and smiled, then said with confidence, "Sir, my name is DD, not nigger. Now, we're going to work together to get you out of this bed and dressed before your family gets here. Since you're not able to do so by yourself, I'm going to help you, alright."

As I was talking to him, my nostrils were flaring out, and my eyes were locked right into his. *Okay, Lord, guide my mind, my tongue, my hands, my heart, my feet, fill me with your holy presence, in Jesus' name, Amen. I'm going to shake it off and help get these people together.*

He replied, "Well, alright then." He began to sit up in bed, and I extended my hand out for him to take hold of it for assistance. Then we carried on with getting him cleaned up and ready for breakfast. We had no more issues with the name-calling afterward.

Yes, people living with dementia say things such as racial slurs, curse words, and derogatory comments. Yet, while it hurts to hear it, they still need help.

I went through the rest of my rooms, assisted everyone out of bed, and gave necessary showers and baths. Passed out breakfast trays and made sure those residents were okay before going to the "ward." When I asked the charge nurse after she gave out assignments what the 'ward' was she replied, "Oh, you'll see."

I took a fifteen-minute break, then returned and told the nurse I'd be in the ward if anyone needed me.

Why does this room smell so bad? Did they assign me to this hall on purpose because I was the new girl? God, I can't do this.

Then I remembered this scripture (Acts 20:35): "In everything, I have shown you that, by working hard, we must help the weak. In this way, we remember the Lord Jesus' words: 'It is more blessed to give than to receive.'"

I gathered the necessary items to provide care for these ladies, but I learned I needed a little more once I started providing their care. The next day, I brought in fragrance for them and shampoo for their hair.

This large old therapy room consists of three beds. One lady's eyes closed shut with mucus-like drainage, her one arm and one leg bearing signs of her battle against an illness that resulted in amputation. Another, her spirit unbroken despite the constraints of her contracted form of both arms and legs, bravely facing the discomfort caused by yeast in every crevice of her body. Her affected skin was inflamed with a red rash, bleeding through cracks, and an extremely foul odor filled the air as you got closer to her. Then, there was a quite spirited lady with hair matted to the back of her head, eyes crusty, her mouth full of gunk, both legs lost to amputation, and a backside of stage 4 bed sores.

I gave them each a thorough bed bath and talked to them throughout the process as they stared at me. Afterward, I fed each of them as they couldn't feed themselves. One was on a puree diet with honey-thickened liquids, and the other two were on a mechanical diet with thin liquids.

At this place, there was a shared shower room for all residents. In order to shower these ladies, I had to get them on a shower bed resembling a stretcher. I locked all the wheels and used the fitted sheet to slide them off the bed and onto the shower bed. I covered them completely to provide dignity, unlocked the wheels, and pushed them down the hall to the shower room.

I showered each lady by myself and cared for them with great attention to detail. As the weeks passed, I assisted with healing their wounds by staying on schedule with keeping them clean and repositioned, and helped to clear out the yeast by keeping the skin folds dry and clean. Even the wound nurse shared how impressed she was with my attention to detail with their care.

I talked to them, and I acted silly even though they couldn't respond to me, but I kept it up. I did receive feedback from them. I counted a smile, a grin, a laugh, and a movement as a positive response to my work with them. These ladies never had visitors. I felt so bad for them. Then I found out they were wards of the state.

I received Employee of the Month within a month of being there. From there on, I was asked to help on the other floors, especially with the memory care unit, which was locked down. I experienced residents screaming while showering, and some were even combative. We kept an extra eye on certain residents because they'd eat things that were not food, such as crayons, tissue, and even feces. One day, I came on to the shift, and a lady had dug feces out of her diaper and was eating her feces. I could not believe my eyes. I suited up with a gown, shoe covers, mask, goggles, and gloves and took her to the shower room on a wheeled shower chair.

In the memory care unit, I learned to keep my head up when providing care, just in case a fist came toward my head or spit shot out of someone's mouth. I always walked through the halls to check on those in their rooms and ensure they weren't getting into mischief. I also encouraged them to do scheduled activities and come up with other things to do outside of planned activities. Then, at mealtimes, I observed those who could feed themselves while feeding those who couldn't.

After all my experience caring for those who need extreme care, the most important thing I want you to know is, it will be hard at times but don't lose faith, pray/meditate, especially when it's challenging.

And I'd like to share some strategies now about bathing and eating.

THE STRATEGY

BATHING

Certain illnesses/conditions, physical disabilities, and mental states can provide a caregiver with challenges. Not everyone will have the same experience because we're all different. What works well for one may not work well for the next. Everyone will experience either providing care for a loved one or the one being cared for. No one is exempt. There are few who make it out of this journey called life not experiencing either. Let's face reality: you don't see people raising their hands to be caregivers. It kind of just falls on your lap whether you're ready for it or not. We take for granted being able to care for ourselves until the time comes when challenges are presented.

I'll provide practical tips that may be a refresher to some or completely new to others, which you can apply immediately as you care for your loved one.

My suggestion would be to have these items listed below in the bathroom before you turn the water on if you are at the point where you have to assist with bathing. It could be a major fall risk if you have your loved one in the shower/bathroom, and then you need to leave the room to gather items.

Bathing may consist of a shower, bath, sponge bath at the sink, or sitting on the toilet (or a bed bath if your person is bed-bound).

Equipment: Shower bench and shower chair on wheels for someone who is a fall risk. If you have a shower where you don't have to step over to get in and you can slide the chair right into the shower, use the Geri shower chair. This is for someone who needs to be laid back a bit to shower; add slip-resistant strips for the floor of the shower to reduce the risk of slipping.

Items needed:

- gloves (if needed)
- three to four towels
- at least two washcloths
- body soap, shampoo, dry shampoo
- lotion
- deodorant
- undergarments-regular or disposable underwear, bra, cami
- shirt
- pants
- socks or TED hose
- shoes
- hair dryer
- comb
- brush
- toothbrush
- toothpaste
- makeup
- shaving cream, razor, or electric shaver
- fingernail/toenail clipper: The best time for nail care is during a shower, this is when the dirt behind the nails softens. Using a manicure stick, clean behind the nails. Then you can clip the nails once they are dressed.

If you don't have the slip-resistant strips for the shower, a small hand towel will work, too. Just hold on to your loved one with both hands. You can also use a gait belt when they move from sitting to standing position from the shower bench. I'd lay a dry towel outside the shower to provide a dry, safe place for the person to step on.

Cover the mirrors with a sheet or the fog from the hot shower water running if your loved one gets angry looking at themselves. They think there's another person in the room, and they don't feel comfortable getting undressed in front of a stranger. I've heard people say with disgust, "Who is that?" when they look at themselves in the mirror.

One common pattern I've noticed over the years of assisting with showers is almost immediately after the shower, a bowel movement takes place. I suggest that after drying their backside, have your loved one sit on the toilet to get lotion on and get dressed. Or you could mention, "Before you get fully dressed why don't you sit on the toilet and make sure you don't need to go."

If your loved one is hesitant about taking a shower and the odor is very strong, you'll need some statements for encouragement. Here are some that I find work well:

- "Maybe we'll go to our favorite restaurant after your shower."
- Share how their favorite person is coming to see them once they've showered.
- "How about a sweet treat afterward?"
- Maybe it's a new outfit to put on.
- "Your pants are soiled with urine; let's take those off. Okay, now let's wash that off of your skin so you don't get irritated."
- Maybe you have to explain that if you don't wash, then yeast can develop, bed sores can develop, and bring on unnecessary discomfort.
- "I promise to leave you alone if you take a shower."
- Maybe they're someone who likes it straightforward, and you just have to say, "You smell like you rubbed manure and raw fish all over you. Let's go wash now!"

Your loved one may mention how they don't want to be cold. You could share that you have a nice warm robe fresh out of the dryer or plenty of warm towels for them in the warm bathroom. As soon as you help your loved one into the shower, be sure the water temperature is comfortable for them. You can also test the water on the back of your hand.

Our skin becomes more sensitive as we age; if you're heavy-handed, please practice washing with a gentle touch. Some of you may experience screaming during a shower. Don't be alarmed or scream back at them. You can try replacing the shower head with a handheld one to adjust how the water shoots out. Some people become scared of the water as their conditions progress. If screaming occurs, in a calm tone, say, "Okay, we're going to go fast so you can get out." I recommend handing them a soaped-up washcloth and encouraging them to start washing underneath their neck, and that usually gets them calmed down enough to complete the shower.

If you're giving a bed bath, ensure you have two wash basins, one for water with washcloths and one for soapy water washcloths. You'll make sure to wash your hands and put on gloves if you choose.

Once you have your loved one undressed, cover them with a warm towel.

If you fold a washcloth in half and then half again, you should have a square. Each side of the fold will be used to clean or rinse the next part of the body.

Wash/rinse/dry the cleanest areas of the body, then move to the dirtiest.

- Eyelids
- Face
- Ears
- Neck
- Shoulder
- Move to one arm, then the other arm.
- Hands
- Chest
- Belly—don't forget the belly button.
- Underneath the stomach, lift up the skin, wash, rinse, and dry—apply anti-fungal powder if it's red and smelly.
- Move to one leg, then the other leg.
- Wash the feet and in between the toes; be sure to dry thoroughly.

- Have them or help them roll over on their side to wash/rinse/dry their back.
- The water will turn cool, so be sure to pay attention to switch out the water in between.
- Use a new washcloth and clean the genital area. For females, you'll need to separate the skin and use a clean side of the washcloth for each wipe. For males, if needed, you'll have to pull the skin back and clean it. Don't forget to fold the washcloth and wash/rinse, using a clean side of the washcloth with each wipe.
- Then wash/rinse the anal area last.
- If you wash their hair with water and shampoo in the bed, you can lay down the big trash bags underneath the pillow to keep the bed dry if you do not have a waterproof protector. Just lay a towel on top of the bag. Or you can use the dry shampoo.

EATING

Certain illnesses/conditions, physical disabilities, and mental states can provide a caregiver with challenges. Unfortunately, as people age, the need to change food and drink consistencies arises.

Oh, the joy of eating food; those of us who experience no problems take this for granted. When I think of eating, this is a time to bring people together. However, as we age, this is a time to pay close attention. Make sure if you're not in the same room with your loved one while they're eating, you have the noise volume low. Keeping a cup of water nearby is a smart move in case choking occurs. Positioning is very important as well, so you want to make sure your loved one is sitting up as straight as possible. If they're lying in bed, please ensure they're sitting up at a 90-degree angle or as close to it as possible. If possible, try encouraging your loved one to eat sitting in a chair.

Some people will notice more drooling and noise while their loved one is eating. If you notice your loved one coughing mainly when eating, call their doctor for a speech therapy evaluation; their food consistency may need to be changed.

I will list diet levels below.

- Regular (cheeseburger with all the fixings).
- Mechanical soft - diet foods are ground up using a Ninja blender (tuna salad without raw vegetables).
- Dysphagia diet - moist, semisolid (canned creamed corn).
- Puree diet - where the food is all at a pudding consistency, no liquid should be able to drain if you tilt the plate (whipped sweet potatoes).
- Nectar thick/honey thick liquids - you can find SimplyThick EasyMix gel thickener on Amazon. It works best if you use a fork to stir in the thickener.
- Thin liquids - hot coffee.

Bob Evans mashed potatoes with the ready-made jarred Heinz gravy is a great go-to. Jack Daniels pulled chicken is great to use as a protein option. Then you'd just need to steam green beans for a quick meal.

If your loved one seems to want to eat all day long, maybe try to add more eggs, oatmeal, cottage cheese, greek yogurt, string cheese, watermelon, spinach, strawberries, blueberries, blackberries, raspberries, carrots, celery, broccoli, and beans to their diet.

Some people will experience their loved ones not wanting to eat. If you place a bowl of ice cream nearby and start with a bite of ice cream first, that may encourage them to open their mouth if you have to feed them. Then, you'd alternate the bites, ice cream, and food.

If your loved one is falling asleep while eating, be sure to have them swallow to ensure nothing is in their mouth. They could aspirate (where it goes down to the lungs and could be the start of pneumonia). Have them take a sip of Coca-Cola. It will definitely help them swallow. Then, let them nap and finish the meal once they have woken up.

If your loved one is living with advanced dementia, I suggest giving them finger foods. The awareness to use a fork or spoon will fade away. You could make stuffed pastries literally for breakfast, lunch, and dinner with different fillings. Cut sandwiches into small pieces for them to pick up. Some may not sit still to eat, so this is another good reason to have finger foods. Or you could offer an Ensure shake for extra nutrition.

If their hands shake while eating, try weighted utensils (available on Amazon). If food slides off the plate, try placing food into bowls or using a divided plate.

I pray those reading this find all of these tips helpful. Make sure to work with your loved one's medical team to provide the proper prescribed care, especially when it comes to their diet.

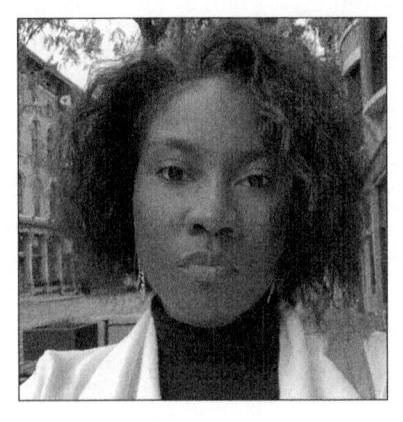

Daneika D. Farmer is the founder of Angelic Sphere, LLC, an early-stage technology for families caring for their loved ones in their homes who are living with dementia. Angelic Sphere will allow individuals, caregivers, families, and healthcare professionals to all be on the same page at all times. Using a wearable device, the platform and connected resources, families can continue to live their busy lives and stay in the know of their loved ones.

Daneika was born and raised in Bowling Green, Kentucky. She learned at a young age how to be a helper for her mother, who gave birth to her sister, and then twins followed a year after her sister was born. Daneika also helped her mom with a family-owned 24/7 child daycare center. She watched her grandmother care for the seniors in her family and picked up nurturing skills from her as well. God has gifted her with a passion for caring for others, and it is definitely in her DNA. Caring for others is her purpose. In 2004, she became a professional caregiver, where she obtained State Tested Nursing Assistant certification. Since then, she hasn't stopped caring for others. Daneika was a hard name for people she cared for to pronounce, so she asked people to call her DD. She worked at a rehabilitation hospital (where people go after surgery), skilled nursing homes, a home health company, hospice, and memory care. She is currently managing the daily operations of a premier 24-bed skilled nursing facility.

She loves to spend time with family, music, dogs, cooking, dancing, cars, having spa days, and being creative.

Connect with Daneika:

Email: angelicsphere1@gmail.com

Website: angelic-sphere.com

CHAPTER 10

The Alzheimer's Conversation

WHY AND HOW TO INCLUDE CHILDREN

Brenda Freed, MMus

MY STORY

"Gran stole my monsters," seven-year-old Olivia sobbed as she ran into the kitchen where Gran and her family were sitting around the table.

"Gran didn't steal them," her mom consoled, patting her daughter's back gently with one hand while flipping the eggs with a spatula in the other.

Olivia withdrew from her mom and shouted, "I know she did!" stomping her foot and turning to look at Gran.

She turned back to her mom.

"They were in my monster box on the coffee table where I showed them to Gran yesterday. Now the box and all the monsters I drew are gone!"

Olivia drew good monsters to help her with scary or challenging situations like electrical storms and homework.

Gran looked confused and sad. She thought, *what's wrong with my sweet Olivia? Why is she accusing me of stealing her monsters? What monsters? I would never do anything to hurt my dear grandchild.*

Alder, Olivia's aunt, suspected Gran's Alzheimer's disease had something to do with the disappearance of the monster box. Olivia had not yet been told about the Alzheimer's diagnosis. It simply hadn't been necessary up to that point because, in the mild stage of Alzheimer's, a person can do almost everything they did pre-diagnosis.

"I'll help you look for your monster box after breakfast," her mom offered. "We'll find it. Now, please, sit down for breakfast."

Olivia plopped herself in her chair and reached for a slice of toast while giving her gran an accusing eye.

Olivia and Gran always had fun together. They loved going for walks, baking cookies, singing, dancing, and playing board games.

I'll search for ways to explain Alzheimer's to children and help repair that relationship, thought Alder.

After breakfast, while Alder searched the internet for resources, Olivia and her mom went upstairs to help Gran pick out something to wear.

Olivia was in the closet and looked down to see her monster drawings scattered throughout Gran's laundry basket. Sure enough, the monster box was there, too.

"I found them! My monsters are in Gran's laundry basket," she yelled in delight with a big smile.

But she wondered, *why did Gran put them in there? That's strange.*

Meanwhile, Alder wasn't having much luck finding resources to help her explain Alzheimer's to Olivia. She'd have to rely on her training in music therapy and psychology to explain how Alzheimer's causes people to do inexplicable things.

The best way to repair the relationship is to get Olivia and Gran doing something fun together, she thought.

Alder went upstairs to where Olivia and her mom sat on the bed, carefully placing the monsters back into their box.

"How about if we all go to the butterfly garden today?" Alder suggested to them, bringing her hands together and folding them as if praying for a positive response.

The response was a resounding "Yay!" from Olivia and "Great idea!" from Gran.

We've made it through that crisis, Alder sighed, giving them two thumbs up.

Alder cared for her mom, Olivia's Gran, for the duration of her Alzheimer's journey, including moving her into her own home for her last three months of life.

In one of our phone conversations seven years after her mom died, Alder invited me to co-create a resource to help families, particularly those with children or grandchildren, to understand and successfully interact with a loved one who has Alzheimer's. She wanted the project to include music and suggested we write a song introducing Alzheimer's disease to children.

Mmm, this sounds like a worthwhile project.

Alder Allensworth and I did our music therapy internships together in 1980. Since then, both of us have garnered a list of publications, presentations, and professional skills. Although my familial experience with dementia is limited to my dad's dying of Covid-induced dementia in 2020, I've always had an affinity for seniors. In high school and college, I worked in nursing home communities. As a music therapist, I worked with geriatrics in memory care and throughout the University of Iowa Hospitals & Clinics. I've performed in residential retirement homes for three decades. In addition, I'm a singer-songwriter.

What a great use of my skills, creating something positive for the underserved children and their families living with dementia.

I accepted Alder's invitation.

I was excited to do some co-creating with Alder. Over the next seven years, we released the Mackenzie Meets Alzheimer's Awareness Program (MMAAP) and the *Mackenzie Meets Alzheimer's Disease Picture Book*. These initiatives, inspired by Olivia's experience with her Gran, provide information, tips, and activities to families living with dementia, particularly those with children or grandchildren. Educating entire families will help people with dementia lead the highest quality of life possible.

THE STRATEGY

WHY AND HOW TO INCLUDE CHILDREN

When I tell people I'm involved with creating initiatives to educate the next generation about Alzheimer's, the first reaction is an unenthusiastic "Ohhhh," as their voices decline in pitch.

That reaction is reflective of the stigma surrounding the Alzheimer's disease diagnosis.

Next, people ask, "Why are you? What are you? Uh, what's your motivation for doing this?"

My thoughts are:

Why wouldn't you want children to know about Alzheimer's and ways to interact with someone who has it?

Why wouldn't you want all people to learn how to maintain family relationships and form positive memories when they're confronted with Alzheimer's?

All these questions lead back to the need for *education*. Alzheimer's is non-discriminating. It can affect *anyone*, regardless of education, socio-economic status, mental health, race, religion, gender, age—even children!

According to the Alzheimer's Association, one in three seniors in the US has some type of dementia[1], the most common being Alzheimer's disease.

There are 2.5 million sandwich generation caregivers: those caring for children *and* for a loved one who has Alzheimer's or any type of dementia[2].

---

1 https://www.alz.org/alzheimers-dementia/facts-figures
2 https://www.ncbi.nlm.nih.gov/pmc/articles/PMC10023280/#:~:text=Results%3A,hours%20a%20month%2C%20p%3D

With baby boomers aging and the occurrence of early onset Alzheimer's on the rise[3], it's highly likely any child could become a caregiver. Rosalynn Carter said, "There are only four kinds of people in the world: those who have been caregivers, those who are currently caregivers, those who will be caregivers, and those who will need caregivers[4]."

I feel passionate about educating children and their families about this disease because it affects *so* many people. The trepidation at the mention of the word 'Alzheimer's' prevents people from reaching out and getting the support they need. It also prevents many with the disease from having meaningful relationships throughout its course, sacrificing their quality of life.

The first step in educating children is to address the big question: What is Alzheimer's disease? To provide an answer that's comprehensible for children yet informative for adults, the *MMAAP* includes a video called *What is Alzheimer's Disease?* As an example of what happens in the brain of someone who has the disease, each step it takes to satisfy thirst is presented: decide on milk, go to the cupboard, reach up, get the glass, go to the refrigerator, choose the milk, and pour the milk. At any step, the brain in someone who has Alzheimer's can get confused and forget what the next step is.

To further demonstrate to a child what happens in the brain of someone with Alzheimer's seeking to satisfy thirst, put a cup of dry cereal in a bowl. Tell the child the cereal represents the person's brain cells. For every step in the task of getting a glass of milk, direct the child to take out a spoonful of cereal. Just as there is less and less cereal in the bowl, point out that the brain becomes less and less able to function properly as Alzheimer's progresses. If most of the cereal disappears before the glass of milk is poured, the person's process of satisfying thirst has been interrupted.

This disruption to thought processes can happen during *any* task. Imagine how frustrating that must be, and then imagine the potential dangers of, for example, forgetting to turn off the stove or getting lost while driving.

---

3 https://www.bcbs.com/the-health-of-america/reports/early-onset-dementia-alzheimers-disease-affecting-younger-american-adults

4 https://www.cjonline.com/story/news/local/2023/01/23/caregiving-part-of-everyones-life-whether-its-giving-or-receiving/69820002007/

The second step in educating children about Alzheimer's is to help them face any fears they have about the disease.

Will Gran and I ever be able to have fun again?

Can I get Alzheimer's disease from Gran?

Will Gran remember me?

Answering their questions will help children feel more comfortable interacting with a loved one who has the disease. Impress upon them that not everyone gets Alzheimer's as they age, and it's not the end of sharing love and happiness with that person.

In the mild stage, the cognitive change is hardly noticeable. Therefore, children can still have fun with their loved ones. However, explain that some activities might need to be modified as the disease progresses. For example, substituting a game of checkers for the usual game of chess might be more enjoyable for Gran post-diagnosis.

Assure children that Alzheimer's isn't contagious like the flu. They can still hold hands and show affection just as they did before the disease. Touch is so important in "promoting overall well-being[5]."

Interactions with a loved one who has Alzheimer's are more likely to be successful when the child (or anyone) always starts by introducing themselves and stating their relationship to that person. For example, "Hi, I'm Olivia, and I'm your granddaughter." It's amazing how this sets a tone of trust with the loved one, indicating that you are someone they know.

Maintaining meaningful relationships across generations is beneficial for most families. However, it's particularly important for families living with Alzheimer's. Connection leads to feeling secure. Children need this connection. But so do people with dementia. You've seen the photos of an older person joyfully interacting with a young child. Connecting with the child helps that person feel needed, instantly providing quality to their life. Preventing the person with dementia from feeling lonely and isolated is crucial.

Sometimes, relationships improve after a loved one is diagnosed with Alzheimer's, but the personality changes resulting from the disease are unpredictable. Sometimes, relationships break down because

---

5 https://eldercarealliance.org/blog/importance-skilled-human-touch-dementia-care/

communication is too difficult: the person with the disease acts angry or mean and pushes loved ones away.

Alder explained to Olivia, "Gran doesn't want to be mean. She has a disease called Alzheimer's that's causing a problem in her brain and making her do things she normally wouldn't do. She needs our love and understanding."

Children who learn about Alzheimer's—the unpredictability of it as well as the expected behaviors—are more likely to respond compassionately when challenging situations arise. This is especially true if they're equipped with an assortment of activities involving music, art, and games to do with the loved one.

Several resources are available that offer a variety of activities children can do with a loved one who has dementia. Access many by searching Google for "free resources for dementia activities." Children who engage their loved ones in activities nurture positive memories with that person, even though the progression of the disease is a difficult journey for everyone.

Children like to feel useful and do adult activities. When caregiving for a loved one who has dementia is divided between children and a responsible adult, it's the perfect opportunity to teach children age-appropriate tasks like folding laundry, feeding pets, tending the garden, washing the car, etc. Recruiting them for some tasks of daily living provides the responsible adult the opportunity to make a phone call, read the newspaper, and practice self-care like meditation, exercise, etc.

Family dynamics change when a loved one receives an Alzheimer's diagnosis. Understanding the disease helps children adapt and prevents resentment when, for example, the daily schedule changes. Bedtime story-reading might get shortened, or the child might need to do more dishes to accommodate mom helping with Gran's evening needs. Resentment can be a new feeling for a child.

Why does Mom have to spend so much time with Gran?

Why do I have to wait before she can take me to see my friends?

Children need their friendships to continue in a normal manner, even though a loved one who has Alzheimer's might be disrupting the amount of time available for friends. It's up to the responsible adult to assure the child they are loved, even though tending to someone else's needs might take precedence.

It's normal for children to feel angry and resentful and to act out. Encourage appropriate expression of their feelings. Talk with them. Listen to them. Help them understand the needs of others. Modeling compassion for what the child is feeling teaches compassion to the child. Designate time in the daily schedule for the child and responsible adult to do an activity or simply spend time together that will give the child needed attention and love.

A sensory deprivation activity is effective in teaching children compassion. Smear some old glasses with Vaseline to obstruct vision. Put cotton balls in their ears to decrease hearing. Place mittens on their hands to decrease their tactile abilities. Instruct them to put their toys and clothes away, make the bed, put on something with buttons or a zipper, and eat their snack while their senses are inhibited.

Remove the glasses, cotton balls, and mittens and talk about how it felt to have vision, hearing, and feeling deficits. Could they remember all they were instructed to do? Explain to them their loved one who has Alzheimer's is experiencing many of these deficits regularly. Once children are aware of what it *feels* like to have Alzheimer's, they are more likely to be empathetic toward loved ones living with it or any other type of disability.

Children experience other emotions when they learn Alzheimer's is changing a loved one.

It's frustrating that Gran repeats herself a lot.

It's embarrassing when Gran needs to be guided to the bathroom in front of my friends.

Encourage children to stimulate conversation with the person by asking questions. They can play detective and try to figure out what the person needs or is trying to express in whatever they're repeating.

To counteract feelings of frustration and embarrassment, teach children to think independently. Provide information and experiences I've described to help them understand their loved one who has Alzheimer's. Rather than worrying about what their friends are thinking, children will have the vocabulary to explain what's happening to their loved one and to express they love them anyway.

Other tips that encourage meaningful interactions with a loved one who has Alzheimer's include the following:

- Maintain a quiet, structured, and familiar environment.
- Encourage interaction with one child at a time.
- Make eye-to-eye contact often.
- Help the person know where they are so they feel safe.
- Teach children when they need to get a responsible adult to help, for example, with bathroom or dressing needs.
- Avoid arguments with the person who has Alzheimer's—no arguing over whose reality is correct.

The ability to tune into others' needs is a useful skill to acquire at a young age. Over time, Olivia learned to adapt to the changes in her gran's behavior. She continued to enjoy time with her gran. But now and then, she knew Gran might do something strange, like put her monster box in the laundry basket. Olivia learned to be understanding and compassionate and offered her gran assistance when needed.

Children exposed to Alzheimer's might be inspired toward certain careers:

I want to become a nurse or physical or occupational therapist.

I want to help find a cure for this ugly disease.

It would be fun to be a music or recreational therapist so I can help people with dementia experience joy each day.

I want to create technology to help people living with dementia.

Approach any discussion about Alzheimer's with sensitivity and openness, using terms children understand. As the responsible adult, be equipped to answer the child's questions. When they ask the difficult ones, that's when they're ready to hear the honest answers. The last thing you want to do is to instill fear in children, reinforcing the stigma you're trying to dismantle.

Breaking down stigmas about Alzheimer's has many benefits for society as well as for families living with dementia. In this time of prevalent and extreme bullying, nurturing inclusivity by respecting everyone, regardless of their cognitive abilities, creates a more sympathetic society. Children educated about Alzheimer's are more likely to be understanding of mental health issues and less likely to fall into bullying roles. They understand how different we all are and how fragile life is.

When is the best time to introduce Alzheimer's to children? The *Mackenzie Meets Alzheimer's Disease Picture Book* comes with the download of the *Mackenzie Meets Alzheimer's Disease Story Song*. The lyrics to the song are the text for the book making the information presentable to toddlers! Included in the *MMAAP* is the animated video for the Story Song. Click this link, https://youtu.be/6d9TbKWFPtM, to show the YouTube video to your children.

Because no cure for Alzheimer's has yet been discovered, it's a disease that's with us and will affect society intergenerationally for years to come. We must do our best to ensure that all who have dementia have access to any cures made available, and will be cared for, treated with dignity, and provided opportunities to live the highest quality of life possible.

The keys to achieving those things are to break down stigmas about the disease, educate children and their families, raise awareness of the prevalence, and share resources available so everyone living with Alzheimer's or any type of dementia is surrounded by love, understanding, and support.

The goal is for children, their families, and their loved ones who have Alzheimer's to continue having meaningful interactions over the course of the disease and to create positive memories.

Here are a few resources offering support and guidance to youth living with dementia in their families:

- https://www.mackenziemeetsalzheimers.com/
- https://alzauthors.com/
- https://www.reminiscencelearning.co.uk/archie

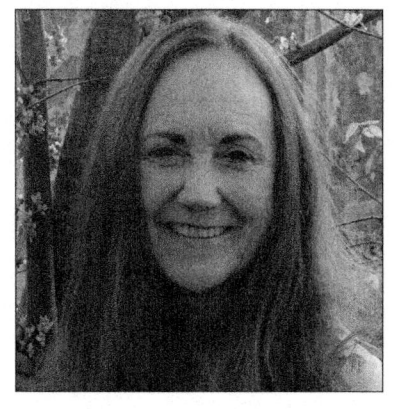

Brenda Freed, MMus, Music Therapy, and Music Education, pioneered the Music Therapy Program at the University of Iowa Hospitals where she worked with all ages and diagnoses, including Alzheimer's.

Freed and Alder Allensworth co-created the Mackenzie Meets Alzheimer's Awareness Program (MMAAP) and co-wrote the song whose lyrics are the text for their *Mackenzie Meets Alzheimer's Disease Picture Book*. Thank you to Alder for sharing her family story that inspired these initiatives.

The MMAAP is digital, multicultural, and includes the following videos:

- What is Alzheimer's Disease?
- Mild Stage Alzheimer's Disease
- Moderate Stage Alzheimer's Disease
- Severe Stage Alzheimer's Disease
- Coping with Alzheimer's Disease for the Responsible Adult with Children

Plus

- Mackenzie Meets Alzheimer's Quick Reference Guide
- Animated Story Song Video & Lyric Video

Written transcripts are offered for the hearing impaired. Because the MMAAP is auditory, it also serves the visually impaired.

Information, tips, and activities for the three stages covered are offered. The video for adults gives tips for talking to children and ways to include them in caregiving.

The *Mackenzie Meets Alzheimer's Disease Picture Book* introduces Alzheimer's to young children. A download of the Story Song is included, making learning fun. The story brings to awareness many aspects of Alzheimer's disease.

A discount code for 50% off the MMAAP is included in the book. Both initiatives are available on the website.

Freed teaches voice, guitar, and piano online, as well as voice and harmony workshops at festivals and conferences. She created and hosts the Young Artist Performance Incubator (YAPI) at the renowned Kerrville Folk Festival. Freed is also a performing singer-songwriter with several published albums of original material. She and her husband perform as Him & Her TX.

Connect with Brenda:

Website & Animated Video: https://www.mackenziemeetsalzheimers.com/

Amazon Book Link: https://a.co/d/bTFGK8S

Email: mackenziemeetsalzheimers@gmail.com

Instagram: https://www.instagram.com/mackenziemeetsalzheimers

LinkedIn: https://www.linkedin.com/company/mackenzie-meets-alzheimer-s/

Facebook: https://www.facebook.com/MackenzieMeetsAlzheimers

YouTube: https://www.youtube.com/@mackenziemeetsalzheimers

CHAPTER 11

Why Did I Come to the Fridge?

FOUR POWERFUL TECHNIQUES TO IMPROVE YOUR MEMORY

Rena Yudkowsky, MSW, Memory Coach

MY STORY

I hate summer camp! I'm not going to camp. Maybe I'll volunteer in the nursing home instead.

That was me at age 16. Thus, I started my 30-year career in gerontology.

Although I didn't know it at the time, that thought was the catalyst that sparked my passion and mission for helping seniors improve their memory.

I signed up to volunteer at Levindale Hebrew Nursing Home in Baltimore, where I worked for the next three summers. I planned and implemented activities, including singing, dancing, and playing word games.

I developed a great love for spending time with seniors. It became very clear to me that I could make a difference in the "depressed and lonely" nursing home resident's life. I was a natural at this, realizing I had what I now call a "Bubby Neshama" or an older soul affinity.

At age 19, when I had to choose a college major, my only interest was gerontology. I specialized in clinical aging and received my Master's in social work a few years later.

My first job was as the director of an Alzheimer's unit in an assisted living facility in Maryland. After I got married and relocated to Israel, I worked in several different part-time positions as I raised my four kids, including a set of twins. I served as the Director of Development for an Israeli senior enrichment program, trainer for professional caregivers, facilitator for caregiver support groups, and memory coach for an anti-aging clinic.

My fascination with understanding the memory process was piqued after working with memory-impaired seniors. When the opportunity arose, I took a memory course after moving to Israel. After years of research and development, I began to teach my memory course for the Geriatric Institute of Yad Sarah. Right before COVID, I decided to offer my memory courses online to reach a wider audience. When COVID hit, I was able to provide stimulating senior programming to individuals and organizations all over the world.

As CEO of Memory Matters, I offer online memory improvement courses for seniors globally and lecture on aging topics internationally.

Grateful that I tapped into my raison d'etre so early on in life, I feel honored to pursue it in such a meaningful way. My mission statement is clear: to empower seniors to feel confident, giving them the tools to believe in their memory skills so they can age with sharper minds.

In addition to my professional experience, I've been learning to use my skills and knowledge to help my family and my husband's family with the challenges of caregiving.

For family caregivers, whether a spouse or a child, the fear of developing dementia is real and tangible. When spending so much time around our loved ones with dementia, we often wonder if it's contagious. Of course, we know it's not, but sometimes it feels like we're losing it. What can we do to improve our memory so we can age more sharply? This is another aspect of self-care that is crucial to consider.

The good news is that we can learn a plethora of techniques and maximize many lifestyle factors to impact the way we age. With increased confidence and tools, we can allay our fears when they become overwhelming.

This chapter will focus on four powerful techniques to improve our memory.

THE STRATEGY

Jim Kwik says, "Your brain is like a supercomputer, and self-talk is the program it will run."

We speak to ourselves about our memory lapses based on our beliefs about our memory abilities, and it is crucial to pay attention to this inner dialogue. If we excuse ourselves, "I can't remember your name, I am bad at names," what message are we reinforcing within ourselves? Is it even worth trying? If we believe that we can't remember names, then what is the chance that we'll remember the name of the next person we meet? Very slim.

But, if we believe that we can remember whatever is important to us, we'll invest the time and energy in learning the techniques, and then we'll have a much greater chance of remembering. Henry Ford said, "Whether you believe you can or you can't, you are right."

Notice what you say to yourself when you forget a birthday. Do you say, "What is wrong with me? I'm such an idiot. Am I getting dementia?" Or do you give yourself time, take a deep breath, and say, "I'll remember this soon, or what technique can I use to help me recall?"

Is our internal conversation demeaning and harsh, or is it gentle, forgiving, and empowering? Which one do you think is going to be more effective for remembering?

What is the connection between focus and memory?

People often say, "I forgot," when they really mean, "I didn't pay attention in the first place." We're not even aware that we're not paying attention to what we're seeing or hearing, and instead, we blame our memory.

The next time you have a "senior moment," ask yourself, "Did I even pay attention to this at all?" This awareness alone can help calm you down. You'll probably realize that you'd have remembered what you wanted if you had focused more.

Do you find yourself walking into a room and wondering why you did it or opening the fridge and forgetting what you came for?

It's a symptom of internal and external distractions that stop us from remembering. You would be distracted if the phone rang while walking to the fridge. If you had many thoughts swimming in your head while walking to the refrigerator, you'd have to rewind your mind when you get to the fridge to help you remember why you went there. But this is not a memory problem. It's a focus problem.

Here are four techniques to improve your focus and a mnemonic to remember them.

TEAS are the keys
- **Task**
- **Environment**
- **Automatically**
- **Senses**

T-TASK

Do one task at a time. That's right, stop multitasking. We're all used to doing many things at once, but it trips up your brain. You might have noticed that as you age, paying attention to more than one thing at a time becomes more difficult. We think we can get away with it when we're younger, but it becomes more challenging and frustrating in our older years.

It's a myth that you're more productive if you do more than one thing at a time. Research done in the workplace proved that people who multitasked made double the number of mistakes, and it took them twice as long to complete the task.[1] Another example of dangerous multitasking is driving while talking on a cell phone, which is the equivalent of driving while drunk. The odds of crashing are four times higher if you're talking on a cellphone and you're half a second slower to hit the brakes![2]

Multitasking can temporarily reduce your IQ by 15 points! It makes you less creative and causes you more stress.[3]

Due to technology, we live in a very distracted world, and we often switch between several windows at a time on our computers. We lose fractions of seconds every time we switch windows. Similarly, switching tasks wastes time. Our brains are sequential processors, which means that we do things quickly but not at the same time.

Living more mindfully means aligning our brains to be present with our bodies. It's a very important part of learning to focus. If I'm talking to my child, but my brain is elsewhere thinking about other things, I can't focus on what my child is saying, and I won't remember that conversation.

This is a real caregiving challenge because we're expected to meet many needs simultaneously. So, wherever possible, ask those demanding of you to wait or be patient. For example, your kids need your attention, but your mom needs to get dressed. Someone has to wait. You have to prioritize and schedule accordingly. You can't do both tasks at the same time.

Often, we feel pulled in different directions, and this stress can damage our cognitive abilities. It's one more reason to practice self-care—to protect your cognition.

A great coping skill is to practice mindfulness, either with deep breathing to feel present or just the visualization of bringing your brain and body into the same space.

Here is a hilarious story that demonstrates this point. My friend was talking to me on her cell phone, and five minutes into the conversation, she said to me, "Rena, you are not going to believe this. I have been looking for my cell phone for the last five minutes!" We had a good laugh, and I explained to her that her mindlessness was the cause of the "forgetfulness."

Other examples include talking on the phone while baking. If you answer the phone while preparing a recipe, you might "forget" the salt! While it's true that certain tasks necessitate less cognition, you have to be careful about details. For example, if you're listening to a podcast while washing dishes (a task that does not take a lot of cognitive power), you might remember the podcast but not all its details.

E-ENVIRONMENT

If you're trying to do a task you want to remember, your environment must be conducive to remembering.

Here are some factors that might affect your focus:

1. Poor lighting while reading
2. Clutter
3. Noise/music in the background
4. Disruptions

If you have trouble seeing, your brain can't encode the information properly, and you'll have difficulty remembering what you read.

If you attend a class or workshop, sit in the front near the speaker. It'll increase your chances of processing the information correctly and remembering it.

A-AUTOMATICALLY

Don't do things automatically without thinking about it. For example, don't throw your keys on the table while thinking five other thoughts. If you do that without engaging your brain, you're not going to be able to find your keys later. Your hand did an action that your brain didn't encode into a long-term memory. Living more mindfully will help you feel calmer and, at the same time, improve your memory.

The only time that doing a task automatically works well is if you have a great system. For example, your keys ***always*** go on the hook by the door. Then, you don't have to waste energy remembering where your keys are because they're always in the same place. It's called a "forget-me-not spot."

Here is an interesting statistic. The average person spends 16 minutes a day looking for lost items.[4] It's so frustrating, yet easily rectifiable.

The best technique for finding lost items (your keys, phone, wallet, glasses) is to pay attention to where you put them at the moment that you put them down. You do this by making the **intention** to remember it and creating a **mental image** that'll pop up in your head when you wonder where you put your keys. The image should be colorful, vivid, funny, action-packed, and exaggerated. You can use whichever image you prefer, but I love a huge bouquet of 100 red roses or a genie popping out of my keys. It only takes a few seconds to create and really works because your mind thinks in pictures.

Hear a piece of information, and you'll remember 10% of it three days later. Add a picture, and you'll remember 65%.[5]

S-SENSES

This one is the simplest and most effective memory hack.

If you use all of your senses to encode the memory, retrieving it will be much easier. According to Richard Mayer's Cognitive Theory of Multimedia Learning, your senses stimulate the brain. If you use one sense to encode a memory, you have a 10% chance of remembering it one week later. But if you use four senses, you are 97% more likely to remember it.

Here are some examples of how you can use this technique to alleviate self-doubt and anxiety related to whether you did these tasks or not.

Did I lock the door?

Look at your hand turning the knob, **feel** the key in your hand, **hear** the clicking sound of the lock working, and **say out loud**, "I'm now locking the door." So later, when you doubt yourself, you will remember hearing yourself say out loud that you locked the door. You can't be on the phone while doing this task if you want to remember it. You need to give it a few seconds of your full attention.

Did I turn off the stove?

Watch your hand turn off the stove, **feel** the knob, **move** the pot to a different burner, and **say out loud**, "I turned off the stove." **Smell** the aroma of what is cooking.

A smell can evoke powerful memories. If you are tested on the details of a movie while the smell of popcorn is wafted in the air, you'll remember 10-50% more.[6]

"Scientists believe that smell and memory are closely linked because the anatomy of the brain allows olfactory signals to get to the limbic system very quickly. Experts say the memories associated with smells tend to be older and thought about less often, meaning the recollection is very vivid when it happens."[7]

I understood this better when I had COVID and lost my sense of smell and taste. It was so confusing and depressing. There was no enjoyment while eating. It was hard to remember what I ate because my brain couldn't process it with the senses of taste and smell.

Did I take my medicines?

Look at the pills in your hand and notice their size, color, and shape. Think about what each one is for. **Taste** them and **feel** them going down your throat with the water. **Say out loud**, "I've taken my Monday morning meds."

Self-talk helps to anchor the memory. A few minutes later, think back to the newly minted memory, which will anchor it even more. Don't worry about people who might think you are crazy for talking out loud. Everyone does it, especially if they are speaking on Bluetooth!

One of my webinar participants shared how this technique improved her quality of life. Every night, she would go upstairs to sleep and then go back down the steps to check if she locked the door. She was frustrated with herself with this nightly waste of time and energy. After I taught her this technique, she used it immediately and no longer had to return to check the door. She felt so good that she could trust herself, remember that she locked the door, and rely on her memory. It was a quality-of-life issue for her, not just a petty nuisance.

So, the next time you think you forgot something, ask yourself, "Did I even pay attention to it in the first place?" If not, use one of these techniques to help you. This awareness alone can help to alleviate the fear of getting dementia.

The quick and simple solution to the "What did I come to the fridge for?" dilemma is to repeat the word "milk" (or whatever you need from the fridge) continuously out loud. At the same time, you walk to the refrigerator to get the milk, not allowing yourself to get distracted by internal or external distractions. This combines the techniques of saying it out loud, staying focused on one task at a time, and being mindful of your tasks.

In conclusion, it is a good thing that I didn't go to summer camp. I have created other **memories that matter** instead.

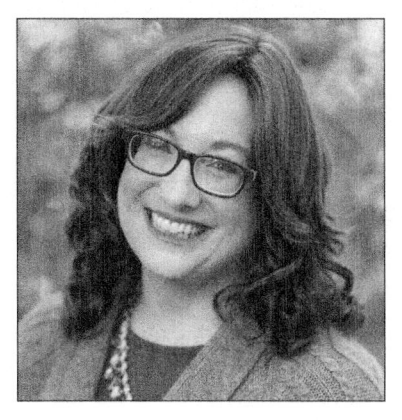

Rena Yudkowsky, a professional memory coach and geriatric social worker, founded Memory Matters. She teaches online memory improvement courses to mid-lifers and seniors. Over the past thirty years in the field, Rena has served as the director of an Alzheimer's unit in an assisted living facility in Maryland, the director of development at a senior enrichment program in Israel, trainer for dementia caregivers, facilitator of support groups, and international lecturer on aging topics. She is a licensed brain health trainer by Dr. Amen, and does 1:1 memory coaching. She is passionate about her mission of helping those 50 + to age more healthfully, both physically and cognitively, as she empowers them to believe in their memory with confidence.

Join her email list and get a free checklist, "Is my memory loss normal?" Go to her website https://www.renayudkowsky.com and sign up.

Links:

Website: https://www.renayudkowsky.com

Email: rena@renayudkowsky.com

Facebook group: Memory Matters-tips and tricks for mid-lifers and seniors https://cutt.ly/memorymatters

You Tube channel: https://www.youtube.com/channel/UC6e-UxB-qTgsjUeHtS2ydrw

Instagram: https://www.instagram.com/renayudkowsky

LinkedIn: https://www.linkedin.com/in/renayudkowsky

Tik Tok: https://www.tiktok.com/@memorymatters

Sources:

1. https://fs.blog/brain-rules-12-things-we-know-about-how-the-brain-works/#:~:text=Smell%20is%20unusually%20effective%20at,than%20those%20in%20unisensory%20environments

2. https://appliedcognition.psych.utah.edu/publications/distractionmultitasking.pdf

3. https://medium.com/@nilssalzgeber/7-reasons-to-ditch-your-multitasking-habit-backed-by-research-7463562cc306

4. American Demographics Report

5. https://fs.blog/brain-rules-12-things-we-know-about-how-the-brain-works/#:~:text=Smell%20is%20unusually%20effective%20at,than%20those%20in%20unisensory%20environments.

6. https://fs.blog/brain-rules-12-things-we-know-about-how-the-brain-works/#:~:text=Smell%20is%20unusually%20effective%20at,than%20those%20in%20unisensory%20environments

7. https://www.verywellmind.com/why-do-we-associate-memories-so-strongly-with-specific-smells-5203963#:~:text=Scientists%20believe%20that%20smell%20and,very%20vivid%20when%20it%20happens.

CHAPTER 12

Be Their Voice

TAKING THE LEAD TO HELP NAVIGATE LATE-LIFE CHALLENGES

Ellen Donovan, RN, BSN, CDP

Despite all its impressive advances, our modern medical system often falls short when caring for older adults. Tip the odds in their favor by being a loud, present, and persistent advocate.

"Strong people stand up for themselves. Stronger people stand up for others."

~ Chris Gardner, Motivational Speaker, Author of *The Pursuit of Happyness*

MY STORY

With her jet-black hair, olive complexion, petite stature, and a personality more befitting someone twice her size, Rita was an old-world Italian woman. She was tenacious, outspoken, and fiercely protective of her loved ones. She was a tough cookie.

But behind all that personality, Rita was among the sweetest, kindest, and most loving people I'd ever known.

Rita was my mother-in-law.

Some of my fondest memories of her are accompanied by the sights, sounds, and smells of a smorgasbord of homemade Italian foods, as might be expected of someone of her heritage. Food was the centerpiece of Rita's life.

Walking into her home, I was captivated by the sizzle of garlic and onion in olive oil, the warmth of freshly baked bread, and the delicious aromas of sweet basil, oregano, and Roma tomatoes congealing into a sinful culinary delight she referred to as "gravy." Her huge meatballs were chock full of freshly grated Parmesan and Locatelli cheese. They were oven-broiled, gravy-finished, and simply melted in your mouth.

"Mangiare" *(man- dza'-re)*, she would say, as she kissed her bunched fingertips in the classic Italian gesture that we all know to mean "delicious." And how right she was!

I remember these meals, not just for the sights, sounds, and smells but for Rita's smile, which didn't leave her face until the last crumb was eaten, the last dish washed, and the last Frank Sinatra song sung.

I couldn't fathom how much time and effort she put into these meals for years, but I now realize it was never really about the food. No, it was about family time, plain and simple.

"I may not have money to give you, but I will always give you my time," she'd say.

That was Rita. To her, the family was everything, and I was every bit a part of that family as were her husband and her two sons.

I think that's why I was so distraught when, at the age of 82, Rita experienced a perforated bowel during a "routine" colonoscopy. This life-threatening situation required an emergency surgery followed by a long, arduous, and complicated recovery. Suddenly, my energetic, larger-than-life mother-in-law was struggling to return to her previously independent lifestyle and survive.

Now, the tables were turned. I always promised to be there if she ever needed me. She always gave me so much of her time. Now, it was time for me to return the favor.

A three-year journey took our family through the whole gamut of late-life healthcare scenarios. My heart dropped into my stomach with the shock of her initial cancer diagnosis. Then came associated chemotherapy, radiation treatments, a messy colostomy reversal procedure, dealing with extended stays at a variety of facilities, and learning to manage in-home care. Ultimately, it was complications associated with a bad fall and shattered hip that ended her life.

The journey was eye-opening, even for a medical professional like me. While I have the utmost respect for doctors, nurses, and the medical community in general and fully acknowledge modern medicine's incredible advancements, I nonetheless found myself repeatedly fighting for Rita as she made her way through the system.

Hospitals made mistakes. Doctors missed things. Staff miscommunicated. Facilities were unsanitary and lacked attention to detail. Sometimes, it felt like nobody cared. If left to fend for herself, Rita wouldn't have survived a month, let alone three years.

I found myself keeping a sharp eye on her condition, questioning every course of treatment, being a part of every decision, and getting comfortable being the "bad guy." I had to be her voice.

In hindsight, this shouldn't have come as a surprise to me. I'd spent most of my nursing career in geriatrics and long-term care, and I'd always noticed that the best outcomes happen when families are most involved. Nevertheless, it got me thinking.

What if I could provide a similar service to others? What if I could be a strong, expert voice for those who need one?

What if I could help prepare aging adults and their families for what might come next and put them in a much better position to handle whatever might come their way?

Such was the genesis of *One Life Consulting*, a boutique consultancy focused entirely on helping older adults and their loved ones navigate the complex world of late-life care.

While working with caregivers and adult children of older adults, my number one piece of advice is almost always the same—*be their voice.* This boils down to three specific actions: observing everything going on, keeping copious notes and records, and communicating thoroughly and persistently with doctors, nurses, and the staff caring for your loved one.

THE STRATEGY

BE THEIR VOICE BY OBSERVING EVERYTHING

When looking out for a loved one who finds themselves in a tricky late-life healthcare scenario, there's absolutely no substitute for being as present as possible and watching and listening to everything that's going on with your loved one and the care they're receiving.

While this might feel like a burden (and it can be), the fact is that the intimate knowledge you have of them is invaluable. You know their tendencies, mannerisms, and behaviors. You know when something looks unusual or different. You know when something is "off" with how your loved one behaves.

Despite all their medical training and caregiving experience, doctors and nurses could never know your loved one the way you do. Thus, your insight can be a critically important part of the caregiving equation, even if those in charge don't outwardly seek your input (and they usually will not).

In these late-life healthcare scenarios, there are two primary aspects of being an observer—namely, paying attention to the course of treatment and how your loved one is reacting to that treatment.

What exactly is being said about your loved one's condition? Is there a specific diagnosis? How confident are doctors and nurses about that diagnosis? Perhaps more importantly, given your intimate knowledge of your loved one, does that diagnosis make sense to you? Trust me when I tell you that your input matters here!

What is the course of treatment? Is your loved one taking medications? If so, which ones, and what are the potential side effects or counterindications of those medications? Have there been, or will there be, any medical tests performed? If so, what are the results, how reliable are those results, and exactly how do those results factor into the diagnosis?

Please know that despite any pushback you may get from hospital staff or caregivers, you have every right to know exactly what the medical professionals are thinking, what they're doing, and what, if any, assumptions they may be making in devising a plan.

You also have the right to make your feelings known if this course of treatment doesn't make sense to you. You have the right to *be their voice*.

In any late-life healthcare scenario, watch your loved one like a hawk. Have you noticed any changes in their appearance or behavior, particularly after starting a new treatment or medication? Adverse reactions can be subtle and escape detection by even the most astute medical professionals. But you know the patient best, and your observations matter. If you notice something, speak up! *Be their voice*.

As a nurse of over 30 years, I've developed a keen sense of when something isn't right with someone. While I'd never expect a layperson to have this same keen sense, I can tell you that much of it comes from simply paying attention, which is something most people don't do.

When you ask your loved one how they feel, look them in the eyes and gauge their response. Do their words match their body language? If they're telling you they're feeling fine but breathing heavily and having difficulty speaking, then they are NOT fine, and you need to escalate the issue immediately.

Again, you know them best. *Be their voice*.

As a poignant example, I recently received a call from a close friend who casually mentioned that she was short of breath when walking up and down stairs, something she hadn't previously experienced. I ran to her house to check on her and immediately noticed she didn't look like herself. She was unusually wide-eyed and pale and nervously rubbing her hands together. When I asked her how she felt, I noticed her response was a bit labored, and she struggled to finish sentences. While she denied any chest pain or tightness, and she tended to minimize the seriousness of her situation, I knew she needed help.

I called 9-1-1, and she was rushed to the hospital, where doctors immediately determined she was having a heart attack and inserted a stent to unblock her coronary artery. She is fine now, but only because she needed someone to *be her voice*.

BE THEIR VOICE **BY RECORDING EVERYTHING**

Helping to manage a loved one's late-life care situation is no small task and requires a surprising amount of organizational effort. One such effort is record keeping, specifically contact management and note-taking.

Most families rely on doctors, caregivers, and hospital staff to update a patient's file with changes in status and important developments in their care. Still, in my experience, too much information gets lost as a patient is passed from doctor to doctor, caregiver to caregiver, and facility to facility.

As ridiculous and disappointing as this may sound, you shouldn't assume that "the system" tracks your loved one's day-to-day progress sufficiently. Thus, you need to do your best to keep track of everything.

Collecting contacts is hugely important to help piece together your loved one's situation later so that you know who to contact if you have questions or need advice.

When you're first introduced to your loved one's attending physician, specialist, or social worker, always ask for their business cards and store them together in a safe, accessible place. Sometimes, these people will act surprised by your question, but most of the time, they'll have their card with them and provide it. A beneficial side effect of the business card ask is that by doing so, you're essentially saying to the medical staff, "I'm here with my loved one, and I intend to be involved." This helps to set expectations and can positively impact the amount of attention your loved one receives. If they can't produce a business card, ask them to spell their first and last name and provide the best contact number for them.

If your loved one resides in a Senior Living Community, ask for a directory of team members so that you'll have this information at your fingertips if you need to contact them.

In addition to storing contacts in a safe place, I suggest you add them to your mobile phone so their names appear when they call you.

You must keep a notebook handy dedicated to your loved one, and amid a crisis, create a daily journal entry. This can be as formal or informal as you want it to be, but be sure to include the date, any test results, a commentary on how your loved one is feeling, a summary of their oral intake for the day (how much they're eating and drinking), what doctors and caregivers are saying, the progress they've made in physical, occupational, or speech therapy, and anything else you feel is important.

This notebook helps to keep everything organized and serves as a great reference tool, both now and in the future. I've realized that we all tend to forget details, especially when under duress, and putting things on paper helps.

BE THEIR VOICE BY COMMUNICATING EVERYTHING

In my practice of helping older adults and their families deal with late-life healthcare situations, poor communication is by far the most significant problem I've seen and the one that leads to most unnecessarily poor outcomes, particularly in hospital settings in which patients are routinely shared between multiple caregivers and an interdisciplinary team of doctors.

If you find yourself or a loved one in such a situation, you simply cannot assume everyone involved during treatment is on the same page. They are required to add notes to the patient's file frequently, particularly when a patient's status changes, but I can tell you that I've seen poorly informed caregivers more often than I can count. So, leave nothing to chance and communicate everything.

It all starts with the intake process, particularly in an Emergency Room. When under duress, older adults tend to miss important facts about their medical history and medications and even tend to miscommunicate, or more specifically, under-communicate the symptoms they're experiencing. I'm not exactly sure why older adults do this, but I've seen it repeatedly in my personal life and practice.

As a point of illustration, years ago, I went to see my 80-year-old grandmother and casually asked her how she was feeling. She responded, "I am okay," in a somewhat faint, quivering voice. I could tell she was trying to be convincing, but I knew something wasn't right. I pressed further and managed to get her to admit that she "Might be a little bit dizzy." I checked her vital signs and found her heart rate to be 38! I called 9-1-1 and had her rushed to the hospital, where they installed a pacemaker that very same afternoon. My grandmother happily lived another 12 years but, according to the cardiologist, would have died that day had I not *been her voice*.

Being the eternal optimist, my mother-in-law Rita was famous for sugar-coating everything, particularly regarding her health. Knowing this, I made sure I always accompanied her to the ER and specialty visits so that doctors didn't get an overly "optimistic" picture of her condition.

I remember taking her to see a nationally recognized surgeon to discuss treatment options for her bile duct cancer. The surgeon's recommendation was to perform on her an arduous procedure called a "Whipple," which I knew would be very rough on her. When I pressed him on Rita's recovery prognosis, the surgeon explained that it would all depend on her ability to tolerate an aggressive rehab, which would involve lots of exercise, including walking long distances every day. He asked her directly whether she could do that, and she replied convincingly, "Absolutely, I walk that much every morning!"

But I knew all too well that Rita could not walk that far, and I made my feelings known, which prompted the surgeon to further assess Rita's actual condition before realizing that she wasn't a surgical candidate. Had I not been a part of that conversation, had I not *been her voice*, Rita and our entire family would have been dragged through a brutal surgery that would have ended her life early.

When speaking with any care team, communicate which medications your loved one takes, any allergies they might have, and even less obvious things like their daily routines, food preferences, and behaviors. For example, they may get agitated in the late afternoon, get up to go to the bathroom three or four times at night, or have a history of falls. Share any information that you think would be helpful for the care team to know about your loved one, even if they don't specifically ask about it. *Be their voice* to help create a safer environment and better outcomes.

When it comes to communication, here's a little industry secret. It always helps to know the "chain of command," particularly in a skilled nursing or hospital situation. Make it a point to assess that early on, especially if you feel like you're getting the runaround. Never be afraid to ask to speak with the person in charge of your loved one's care. In skilled nursing facilities, this might mean the Director of Nursing or the Community Administrator. This might mean the physician in charge of the case in a hospital setting. I know it takes courage to do this, and it won't help you make any friends, but it can save your loved one's life. The tougher the situation, the more you need to step up and *be their voice.*

BE THEIR VOICE **BY BEING THEIR ADVOCATE**

The suggestions I've provided here: observing, recording, and communicating may seem obvious and oversimplified, and conceptually they might be. But the one thing they have in common is that they all require you to be their advocate (and a relentless one).

Advocating for an aging loved one means being there for them (physically, mentally, and emotionally). It means ensuring they never feel alone and that they're heard when they need to be. Perhaps most of all, it means being willing to fight for them when nobody else does.

There's nothing easy about any of this. Advocating for an aging loved one can be one of life's most difficult, frustrating, and flat-out exhausting challenges. If and when you find yourself in such a situation, please try to find some solace, knowing that you're doing your best. Know in your heart that you're giving of yourself to ensure that your loved one receives the best care possible. In life, there may be nothing more admirable.

Love them. Advocate for them. *Be their voice.*

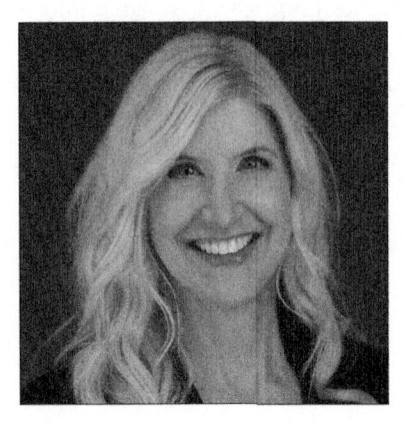

Ellen Donovan is an RN Senior Care Consultant, Certified Dementia Practitioner, and President of *One Life Consulting*, a boutique consulting firm that helps older adults and their families navigate the many challenges associated with late-life care, including late-life care planning, patient advocacy, aging in place, community selection and placement, and crisis management. Ellen has devoted her entire 30-plus-year nursing career to providing the best outcomes for older adults. She now brings this expertise to the senior care community in a new and unique way.

Ellen is an ambassador for the Eastern Montgomery County (PA) Chamber of Commerce and proudly supports several altruistic causes. She is a proud captain of the *Walk to End Alzheimer's* in Philadelphia, an event she looks forward to every year.

She also publishes a free monthly email newsletter called *Sustenance* that is devoted entirely to self-care, something she believes applies to everyone, regardless of age or life situation.

Ellen is a health and wellness enthusiast and eagerly shares her knowledge and best practices with others. She enjoys spending free time at the Jersey shore with her family and short-legged, long-eared, very stubborn basset hound Fred.

Connect with Ellen Donovan:

Website: www.onelifeadvocates.com

Facebook: www.facebook.com/OneLifeAdvocates

LinkedIn: www.linkedin.com/in/ellen-donovan

Twitter: www.twitter.com/Ellen_OneLife

CHAPTER 13

A Different Feel

NAVIGATING DEMENTIA SENSORY CHANGES WITH EASE

Kim Kasiah, PAC Certified Trainer, Coach, and Champion Teacher

MY STORY

A few years ago, I suffered a traumatic brain injury that changed my life. A TBI is not the same as dementia, while some effects seem very similar.

At the time, I was working with families and loved ones to navigate senior living care and taught dementia training classes throughout the state. My grandma introduced me to dementia over 20 years ago, and I have dedicated my life to building a better understanding of it.

Everything changed for me overnight. My blood pressure was out of control, and standing up quickly made me dizzy, falling headfirst onto a metal heater. I was knocked unconscious and suffered a severe concussion. The effects lasted for over a year before I could function again.

My speech was the most noticeable change. Stuttered mumbles of sounds, no understandable words came out. Writing down messages helped, but spelling was a struggle. When I focused too hard, stabbing pains went through my head, making me nauseous. I used hand gestures to communicate, but it wasn't the same as talking.

If someone was speaking, I could only focus on one thing at a time. With questions, I processed the first one while they were on the fifth. It made it easier if they spoke slower and paused so I could process, but very few people did. Frustrated with my garbled speech, I slammed my hand down on the table and walked away. I wasn't angry with the person talking to me, just myself. I recalled when residents made similar actions and how they were perceived. Perhaps we had gotten it all wrong.

Lights and sounds made my brain come to a standstill, and I couldn't think or make a sound as the pain went through my head. My hearing became very sensitive, and certain sounds, like vacuum cleaning, caused a seizure, which I hadn't experienced previously. I wore earplugs and sunglasses constantly to reduce my exposure. Watching TV or working on a computer or cell phone was out of the question.

My family wanted to help me, but no one knew how. I didn't either. I overheard conversations about my future if I didn't recover, making me feel like a project that I had no input on. It didn't feel like my life anymore. I wondered if I'd made someone feel like that while trying to help them and their families figure things out.

I thought about the past me. I used to move crowds to silence, tears, or laughter with my words. My favorite hobbies were going to concerts and playing old-school video games. I taught classes and answered questions in the moment. Those abilities were gone, and this stranger who looked like me took over instead. This stranger could barely take care of herself, let alone others.

For many years, I taught that we all have value, regardless of our limitations. We just needed reminders at times.

My reminder happened when I discovered a man face down on the sidewalk. Turning him over, he was cold to the touch, blue with no pulse. Two other men joined me as we started CPR and called 911. At this moment, I knew what to do while we worked tirelessly on him. His pulse would come back and be gone again. We worked for six minutes until paramedics arrived, shocking his heart there in the street. He suffered a widow-maker heart attack. I learned the next morning that Steve, the 49-year-old man, survived without brain damage. It was a miracle that he was alive, no less without damage to his brain.

It wasn't lost on me that without my TBI, I would've been sitting at my desk working. I was able to help someone even if my speech and processing were different than before. It showed me I could still make a difference and needed to focus on everything I could still do instead of what I couldn't—just like what I was taught in classes. The change in my perspective helped a lot. I had to take it slow and not be so hard on myself because that attitude made recovery feel out of reach.

Eight months later, I taught my first class in almost a year.

Five years later, I'm able to do most of the things I used to do, including going to concerts again! I savor the moment instead of rushing to the next. Since then, I've earned two additional certifications from Teepa Snow's Positive Approaches to Care dementia program and worked at a Memory Care during COVID with 42 individuals with mid to late dementia as Life Enrichment. I understood my special friends living with dementia more than ever, and I'm thankful for the insight my injury taught me.

THE STRATEGY

We often get so focused on the differences that happen with dementia that we forget to look at the person who still lives and see the changes instead. I made that mistake with myself.

Education has always been the key for me, and the experiences taught me even more. Since I lived with sensory changes, I felt it was time to share my story along with how the five senses play a big part in our lives and our person living with dementia.

The five senses (visual, verbal, touch, smell, and taste) allow the brain to absorb information while developing preferences, making us each an individual. A healthy brain processes at such lightning speed it can be taken for granted how amazing it is.

After the mid-20s, the brain's processing ability will gradually slow. Since it's such a powerful and complex processor, we normally don't notice until we are in our 40s that we're taking more time to think and respond. We walk into a room, forgetting why we had come there. Backtracking and retracing our steps is a normal part of aging.

Developing dementia increases with age while not a normal part of the aging process. Dementia is a progressive disease affecting many functions, such as memory, language, and cognitive ability. It changes many parts throughout the brain and body.

Dementia changes the sensory system in which the senses are felt, processed, and expressed. It can create confusion for the person living with it and those providing care.

THE VISUAL SENSE

Our vision system contributes the largest amount of sensory input to the brain of the five senses. It's an example of the "we have to see it to believe it" concept.

The person living with dementia pays closer attention to what is seen rather than heard. Sometimes, they'll mirror what's seen. If you're smiling, they will probably smile too.

The visual field or peripheral shrinks with the progression of dementia. In early-stage dementia, visual changes become like wearing a scuba mask constantly. During the middle stage, this changes to looking through a set of binoculars, only able to focus on one place at a time. In the late stages, the brain turns off one eye, and vision becomes monocular. All of these factors will change depth perception, causing accidents or falls.

Visual changes with a changing processing center require a slower approach. Approaches should be from the front. Never from behind or the side as it can startle someone, triggering the fight, flight, fright, or freeze part of the brain.

The goal of the approach is to get the person's attention with visual cues such as a slight wave around the face. Start six feet in front of them. If they're looking down get to their level to get their attention. Offer a handshake to build connection. Moving slowly towards their dominant side, give a verbal greeting while turning sideways instead of squared up in front of them. The person can see past you and not be confined by your body position. When next to them, get to their eye level or slightly below, keeping your body sideways.

As you move through your approach, observe the body language to get information about them. Abrupt changes can signal pain or agitation. Backing off and trying something different might be necessary. Take three deep breaths when stressed to calm yourself and help your brain think more clearly. The person with dementia may mirror you doing deep breathing and become calm, too.

Use gestures to provide extra cues.

In the early and mid stages of dementia, write short messages to help communicate. As the disease advances, reading ability can be lost.

The color black may be perceived as a hole, and some will walk around it while others avoid it completely.

If the person with dementia suffers from an eye disease, know that effects on vision, such as cataracts, can increase the glare from lights, making vision cloudy while decreasing color brightness.

For glasses wearers, clean lenses often by running under slightly warm water while applying dish soap. Dry using a soft cloth. Swab alcohol on the nose pads and temples. Check for sores on the nose or ears. Inspect lenses and frames for scratches, breakage, and adjustment, especially after falls. Most eye care professionals offer adjustments, repairs, and fresh nose pads.

AUDIO/HEARING SENSE

Hearing sounds is the second largest input.

The brain must perform many steps when we have conversations. We have to hear what is said, keep track of the information along with tone, processing the content while forming a response.

Hearing loss affects about one-third of adults age 60 or older.

The loss of hearing can be caused by loud noises, high blood pressure, diabetes, heart issues, and strokes. Medications, ear infections, and build-up of ear wax also decrease hearing. The chance of hearing loss increases with age.

Untreated hearing issues cause the brain to work harder to compensate, causing a higher risk of developing dementia. Hearing impairments can also lead to social isolation, depression, and less cognitive stimulation.

An audiologist helps determine the cause of hearing loss, which may be improved with hearing aids, implants, or surgery. The hearing device needs to be fitted and cleaned regularly.

Dementia changes the ability to produce speech and comprehension of words. One out of four spoken words are lost by a person living with early-stage dementia. By the middle stage, two of four words are dropped. Talk slower with fewer words while using gestures and facial expressions, pausing to give time to process. Demonstrate the tasks that you want your person to do. The tone of voice conveys the emotion of the message. The person notices the tone and facial expressions rather than the words spoken.

As dementia progresses, the ability to produce speech changes. In the early stage, words might be replaced with others that don't make sense. In the mid-to-late stage, words can become mumbled or mashed together in a word salad. Sometimes, our person vocalizes sounds instead of words as it's easier.

Care providers can use rhythm with their person. A song or rhythmic phrase such as "Up! One, two, three, four" with a gesture to stand up can work better than words. The retention of rhythm in the brain is how a person with advanced dementia can sing a song they are familiar with. Music, poems, prayers, and rhymes can be helpful in the mid and late stages of the disease.

TOUCH SENSE

With a healthy brain, you can touch a hot surface and decide if it's safe to touch or should move away quickly. You can feel pain, convey it, and show the location.

Dementia changes the sensation of touch throughout the body. Most physical sensations become lost while four parts of the body retain sensitivity: The hands (especially the palms and fingertips), the mouth and lips, the feet (primarily the soles), and the genitals. These areas can become hypersensitive.

By mid-stage, the person will use their hands to explore surroundings by touching walls and objects, taking items if they like the sensation. Make the area safe to explore as safety awareness is lost. They can benefit from sensory activities. Offer different materials, textures, and colors that can be folded, stacked, or sorted. Include items that were used in past professions or hobbies, like an adding machine or an old camera. Fidget boards or mats offer many sensory items in one place.

The person still experiences the sensation of pain while unable to tell the location or severity of it. A change in behavior often affects how pain is expressed. Unfortunately, we may not notice their cues or behavior differences overlooking the message. Use your approach and observations to investigate changes. It can be hard to look past behavior challenges and remain objective to the communication presented. It can take an investigation to figure it out.

SMELL SENSE

Ever wonder why smells take you back to childhood? Breathe in cinnamon, and suddenly, you are standing back in your grandma's kitchen, being taught how to make an apple pie.

The sense of smell is very powerful.

It's designed to keep us safe and help us find food while alerting us to danger. The smell of smoke can alert us to a fire. Food with a bad odor will tell us that it's spoiled and not safe to eat.

Babies are born with the ability to smell, and the sense grows with us. Many smells were encountered for the first time during childhood, becoming linked with the memory.

When consuming food, the smell of it can rev up the taste buds. Walking into a room with food cooking may cause your stomach to start growling.

Dementia diminishes the smell sense, which can lead to a decrease in appetite. Sometimes, our people aren't aware they're experiencing a decrease in smell. Scented oils or aroma therapy can help, as these scents are usually stronger. Flowers that are non-toxic with a strong smell, such as roses and lilacs, can be beneficial.

TASTE SENSE

Imagine eating your favorite meal cooked to perfection and savoring each bite. You experience different flavors with just the right spices to accent. Just when it seems that it can't get any better, out comes your favorite dessert from that wonderful little bakery.

Think about the flavors. What did you taste?

The sense of taste gives us the ability to enjoy different flavors. There are five taste types: sweet, salty, sour, bitter, and savory.

Health issues such as strokes, diabetes, cancer, kidney failure, and COVID, along with smoking and alcohol, can change the sense of taste.

Dementia changes the taste senses with sweet and salty remaining throughout the disease. With diminished taste, the person can experience weight loss as they may not like the food any longer. They might oversalt their food to make it taste better or eat only sweets, which make it challenging to provide a healthy diet. Try using honey or sweet potatoes to make food taste sweeter.

Remember to look at the person behind the diagnosis and educate yourself. There may be many wonderful ways to help them with the sensory changes they've experienced so that they can thrive.

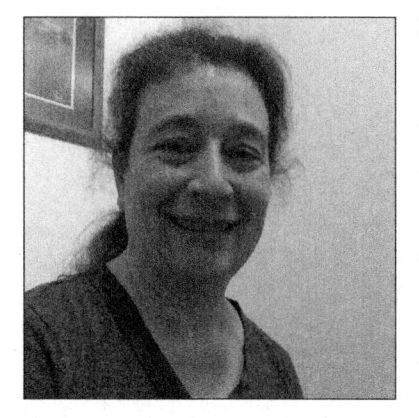

Kim Kasiah has lived in Southern Oregon all of her life. The first person to teach her about dementia was her beloved grandma, and she never forgot what it felt like to be an overwhelmed family member while trying to make sense of the changes that dementia can bring. In 2013, she left a 20-year career in the optometry field to pursue working in the senior care industry as a marketing director at an assisted living to follow her passion for helping and working with older adults and their families. The following year, she founded a family member/caregiver support group through the Alzheimer's Association in Grants Pass, Oregon, and continues to facilitate it ten years later.

Kim has worked with over 1,500 individuals living with dementia along with their families.

Teaching dementia education classes on behalf of the Alzheimer's Association since 2014, she found education was the key to understanding and unlocking many of the mysteries of this confusing disease. In 2016, Kim became a Certified PAC Dementia Trainer through Teepa Snow's Positive Approaches to Care® (PAC™) program and, later, a Certified Dementia Coach to help the caregiver apply the training to the individual and situation. In 2023, she received her third certification as a PAC Champion Teacher to offer advanced training and skills to caregivers and families. She has been a trainer for Oregon Care Partners since 2016, in addition to the Alzheimer's Association, long-term care facilities, adult foster homes, and families. In June 2023, she was honored to teach alongside her longtime mentor, Teepa Snow, the founder of Positive Approaches to Care (PAC).

CHAPTER 14

Finding the Gift

WHEN CAREGIVING HAS NO END IN SIGHT

Diane Marie Gallant

It's not the load that breaks you down, it's the way you carry it.

~ Lena Horne

MY STORY

I felt like I was hit by a high-speed train.

How can I possibly take care of my two parents all on my own?

As an only child I knew the responsibility of caring for my parents would one day be mine. In an instant, the task of caregiving was thrust upon me just days after my 30-year marriage ended. A foreboding sense of burden lurked in the background.

I never saw it coming.

Family has always been important to me. I included Mom in all the big events.

After my daughter was engaged, she lined up three bridal boutique appointments to shop for wedding dresses. Mom and I anticipated this day for months, eager to witness my daughter's *"Say Yes to the Dress"* moment. Finally, this exciting and significant day arrived. I was filled with joy.

My daughter and I were out the door when the phone rang. It was my mother.

"Diane, I hate to tell you this, but I won't be able to meet you." I'm alarmed and brace myself.

"Why not, Mom? What's going on?"

"Yesterday, I started seeing white flashes out of the corners of my eyes and feeling off. I don't think I can drive."

My heart drops. Instinctively, I know something bad has happened.

"Why didn't you call?"

"I didn't want to concern you and hoped to feel better today. I was *really* looking forward to wedding dress shopping with my granddaughter."

After a flurry of phone calls, one of my parents' neighbors offered to bring Mom to the hospital where she was immediately admitted.

I wish I could be in two places at the same time! I'll take lots of pictures for Mom.

The next day, we receive the tragic news: "You had a cerebral hemorrhage."

We were stunned.

Mom looked so fragile lying there in the hospital bed. Turning away, I wiped my tears. *I have to be strong for all of us. My mother's life will never be the same.*

And then it hit me: **My life** *will never be the same!*

Nothing about this journey will be easy.

Mom moved to a rehab hospital and stayed for a month to work on her balance, adapt to peripheral vision loss, and gain her strength back. It was likely she'd never drive again.

Since my father was legally blind and had signs of dementia, I moved in to take care of him. I was alarmed by the extent of his forgetfulness.

He frequently asked, "Where is Dot?" and couldn't remember if he took his pills. *Does Dad have Alzheimer's?*

I expressed my concerns to Mom, but she couldn't face it. She had too much on her plate to take this in. When she returned home to care for Dad, I moved back to my house.

After months of testing, we finally met with a neurologist to get her MRI results. We sat in the exam room nervously chatting, waiting for him to come in.

The door swings open, and our conversation immediately ends.

As the doctor sits across from Mom, he reaches out to hold her hands. I see both compassion and anguish in his eyes. *It's bad news.*

"I'm very sorry to tell you this, but we found brain tumors. There is also a suspicious mass in your liver. We need to do more testing."

The room begins to tilt and the air feels thin. *Did I hear correctly? This can't be happening. I can't bear the thought of losing my mom. I want more time with her!*

Tears immediately stream down my face. Turning toward my mother, I see her sitting there stoically as she receives this terrifying news. My heart breaks for her.

At the next doctor's appointment, bad news keeps coming. "We have the results from your liver biopsy. The source of your cancer is malignant melanoma."

The melanoma that was removed from her back thirty years ago had returned. Mom had Stage 4 cancer.

This is devastating! I must reassure Mom I'll be with her—every step of the way!

She was facing a long and arduous road ahead of her, and so was I.

Committed to helping, I jumped into action. Since she could no longer drive, caring for both parents would fall completely on my shoulders. Even though I was a born nurturer, the responsibility of caring for two aging parents single-handedly was daunting and, honestly, not something I looked forward to.

With shock, I realized I exchanged one set of stressors for another: There would be no time after my divorce to regroup and collect my energy.

Juggling my parents' steady stream of doctor appointments, household duties, meals, and laundry, all while learning to live on my own, weighed heavily on me.

I grumbled to a friend, "My caregiving journey has barely begun and I'm already feeling stressed and overwhelmed. I feel like a walking time bomb!"

"Don't be so hard on yourself. Look at everything you're accomplishing. You're doing a great job!"

I only saw what I wasn't doing.

My inner critic was relentless and discouraging. *You're doing a terrible job managing your life. Look at those dirty dishes in your sink and smell the stinking cat poop near the litter box. Your life is a disaster. GIVE UP!*

I crumbled under the weight of self-judgment.

Right after Mom's chemotherapy treatments ended, she had another cerebral hemorrhage. Although her mind remained sharp, she was left weaker than before. Again, she was admitted to the rehab hospital for another long stay, and I was back living with Dad for the second time.

His faculties had noticeably declined, so I brought him to a geriatric psychiatry clinic for evaluation. My suspicions were confirmed.

"Your father has advanced Alzheimer's Disease."

*You've got to be kidding me! I can't take anything else on. I'm only **one** person!*

When Mom moved back home after her rehab stay, both parents were placed on hospice care. Even though this provided some emotional relief, my mood remained dark. I *desperately* needed a break.

I decided to go on a sacred trip to Peru to lift my spirits and soothe my soul. I worried about leaving Mom alone with Dad because she was weak, and he needed a lot of assistance. His rapid weight loss was also concerning, but hospice reassured me they'd both be fine. I lined up home care for them, took a deep breath, and left.

At the end of the trip, my daughter called. "Pepe is not doing well and Meme said she can't take care of him much longer. What should I do?"

"Call hospice right away and ask for some support. And *please* try not to worry. I'll be home in two days."

I can't believe Dad is going downhill so fast! I shouldn't have gone on this trip.

At 5 AM the next morning, the phone rang. It was my mother. "Diane, I'm very sorry to tell you this, but your father died last night."

I was instantly slammed with anguish as my greatest fear came true.

Dad, you weren't supposed to die while I was away!

Riding home on the bus from the airport, my pen jumped up and down as I wrote his eulogy on scraps of paper. I breathed deeply in an attempt to relieve my overwhelming feeling of grief. It was an exhausting ride home.

Now that Dad was gone, I was concerned about Mom living alone. I wanted to preserve her independence as long as I could. I went back and forth between our homes for a year, bringing my senior cat with me for overnights. As if that weren't enough, the COVID-19 outbreak added even more stress to an already pressure-filled situation.

I can't keep rushing around continuously with little to no rest for much longer! Maybe it's time to sell Mom's house?

It was gut-wrenching to consider parting with our family home. My parents built this house when I was a toddler and we had a lifelong history there.

I asked my mother what she thought. "Do what is easiest for you, Diane. I will adjust."

The decision was made. We sold her home, and she moved in with me.

I exquisitely attended to Mom's every need. Things were going very well for her, but I was quietly falling apart.

My personal life was at a standstill. I quickly blamed my caregiving responsibilities for taking away my spontaneity, time with my first-born grandchild, long hikes in the woods, fun with friends, chill-out time, and building a career.

Psychologically resistant to the truth of my reality, my mood was spiraling downward. I was despondent, hopeless, and frustrated.

I can't move forward in life because I'm trapped by caregiving responsibilities. There's no end in sight!

Then, the realization hit me.

My mother isn't the one holding me back in life. I am!

It was *my choice* to step into this caregiving duty. I volunteered to do this out of love for my parents. They were not to blame. It was time to get off this negative path for *both* our sakes.

It took hitting rock bottom before I could see things in a new light.

I don't need to wait until Mom moves out to take steps toward a new life and career. I can start now!

It was my turning point.

When I permitted myself to slow down, I could see more clearly. I learned to live in the present moment, which helped me to be more patient and loving toward my mother. I also began prioritizing myself and scheduling time during the day to rest and have fun. These shifts helped me to become a better daughter—*and* a better caregiver.

A close friend reminds me, "Enjoy the freedoms you have." He's so right!

Rediscovering the simplest things, like listening to rainfall, brings feelings of peace and gratitude deep into my heart. This focus helps me to see the multitude of tiny treasures that have been waiting for me all along. Finding these gifts fills my empty spaces and brings me back toward wholeness.

When I made this transition, a newfound vigor flooded in.

My healing had begun.

This is moment-by-moment work. Some days are easy—and others are hard.

Reflecting on my caregiving journey, I find so many unexpected gifts. Sharing quality time with Mom has brought us closer. I learned that "good enough" can be great, simple pleasures are within reach, and I even have time to squeeze in online classes to advance my career.

My mother naturally lives in a state of ease and flow. I joke with her, "You're ruining it for me! I'll never be as good as you!" Her eyes light up with the ownership of knowing who she is and how she positively impacts others.

My mother is truly one of my greatest gifts. I'll carry on her exceptional legacy of kindness and compassion and look back on our time together without regret. I will miss her terribly when she is gone.

With clarity, I see caregiving as an unpredictable journey that holds many opportunities for personal growth and discovery.

I've learned that changing my perspective from burden to balance is possible. Allowing my higher self to expand my vision through meditation and prayer reveals new possibilities. Life feels hopeful again and even exciting at times!

Always remember *you* deserve to receive the same exquisite care that you give. The more you give to yourself, the more you'll have to give to others—and the better equipped you'll be to conquer caregiving challenges.

Your loved ones are counting on you!

THE STRATEGY

All caregivers experience stress. It's par for the course. This isn't a job you can prepare for in advance. It's learned by juggling endless demands. Stepping into this role will challenge and stretch you in ways you can't imagine—and radically change your life.

There are two ways to cope with stress. You can choose to do nothing and continue to let the weight of the experience crush your spirit and potentially affect your health. Or you can pivot and discover a way out as I did.

Here is a strategy that helps me manage the demands and stresses of caregiving.

ASSESS YOUR STATE OF BEING

Because your thoughts, emotions, and actions are indicators of your inner state of being, it is vital to slow down and evaluate your feelings.

If you notice your feelings are plummeting, please check in with yourself to see what is going on. If you don't, you run the risk of burnout.

<u>Begin by asking yourself:</u>

- Am I at peace or am I flustered?
- Am I grieving the loss of my independence and former lifestyle?
- Are my thoughts helping or hurting me today?

Let these answers inform you. Avoid labeling your feelings as good or bad, and drop any judgments toward yourself, others, and circumstances. Judgment only adds more pressure to your day.

BROADEN YOUR PERSPECTIVE WITH BREATH

When I'm overwhelmed, everything feels like one giant problem. When this happens, I know my emotions have taken over and are calling the shots, keeping me in a state of depletion.

If I'm having a good day, I can break challenges into smaller parts and tackle them one at a time. Seeing progress helps me feel accomplished, which supports my overall mood.

However, sometimes, I'm gripped by negative emotions that are hard to shake off. When I feel this way, I use a breathing technique I learned from my Positive Intelligence® coaching program. It helps me to "zoom out" from my problems and connect with a broader perspective so I can find creative solutions.

Let me guide you with this breathing exercise. It is a great tool to reduce your overall stress.

<u>Breathing exercise:</u>

Begin by closing your eyes and focusing on your breath. Next, gently rub two fingertips together on one hand while feeling all the ridges on the tops of your fingers. Notice all the sensations of touch. Breathe.

Now, be aware of the temperature of your breath as it enters and leaves your nostrils. Breathe.

Next, listen to the furthest sound away, then slowly shift your attention to the sound of your breath. Breathe.

If your mind drifts, return your focus to the sensation of touch, the rhythm of your breath, or the sounds around you.

Bask in the present moment, and allow feelings of peace and relaxation to come in. Breathe.

Connect with your inner wisdom.

<u>With curiosity, ask:</u>

- Why am I upset?
- Is there a different approach I can take to address this problem?
- What opportunities do these challenges present?

Allow time for your higher self (the loving, intelligent part of yourself that knows what is best for you) to answer. Don't rush the process. Listen, watch, and be open to receive insight.

Stay in this state of contemplation for as long as you need. As you relax, you will notice stress melting away. When ready, slowly open your eyes and return to the room.

Doing this breathing exercise for two minutes, at least three times a day, promises to create new mental habits to improve your overall well-being, relationships, and productivity.

Listening to the whisperings of your heart and intuition will spark your inner light and bring forward supportive new perspectives designed just for you!

For an audio version of this experience, go to:

https://dianemariegallant.com/meditations/caregivers-advocate/

PRACTICAL STEPS TOWARD WHOLENESS

Finding ways to feed your *whole self* (body, mind, and spirit) will improve your outlook, increase your energy, and help you become a better caregiver.

Eating healthy food, drinking plenty of water, exercising, and getting enough sleep are the foundations for everything you do. *These steps cannot be overstated!*

I enjoy spending time with my family, walking outdoors, and tending my garden, which support my overall well-being.

Meditating, reading spiritual books, journaling, and connecting with energy healing feed my soul.

I also allow my inner child to "come out and play" so she can be silly and lighthearted. This lifts my mood by reminding me not to take things so seriously.

Adding variety to life helps stave off boredom for you and your loved one. Try visiting new places, playing different card games, or watching a newly released movie. And ask them for their input. They may have ideas and desires that will surprise you!

What steps can I take:

- What do I need most right now?
- Can someone help me? Or should I hire help?
- Is now a good time to reach out for coaching or professional support?

Choose an action that will refuel you and follow through. You'll see how positivity grows when you take steps to support yourself.

* * *

Your personal life still exists. It only looks different.

By finding the gifts within your circumstances and enjoying the freedoms you have, you can still thrive within the responsibilities of caregiving.

Remember, prioritizing yourself is a loving act, not a selfish one. Your loved ones benefit when you are rested and happy.

Your caregiving journey is a meaningful act of service that will provide you with personal satisfaction and cherished memories. Praise yourself for stepping into this role, and keep your spirits up.

You got this!

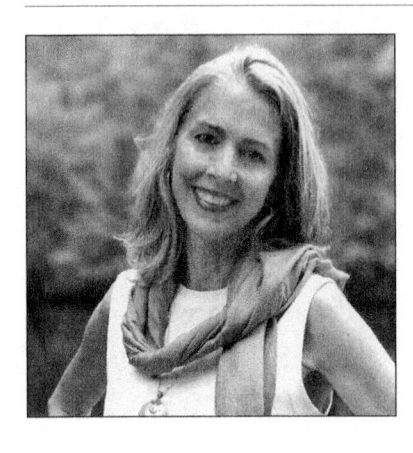

Diane Marie Gallant is a Mental Fitness Coach, Reiki Master Teacher, and Death Doula.

Diane lives in New Hampshire and offers mental fitness coaching with energy healing support. She works with individuals and groups both in-person and online. She also teaches certified classes and workshops.

As a highly intuitive and natural-born healer, Diane creates an environment of safety and trust. She empowers her clients to believe in themselves and develop supportive habits to thrive.

She has been coaching and empowering clients for over 15 years and is certified in many healing modalities. She is completing her Positive Intelligence® and Doulagivers Institute™ certifications. Her BS degree in the medical field adds to her broad knowledge base in health and wellness. Trauma, stress, and nutrition are other areas of expertise.

Her neuroscience-based coaching helps clients identify sabotaging patterns that interfere with their lives. Clients are equipped with easy-to-learn mindfulness tools to reinforce a positive mindset and lasting change.

Energy healing helps her clients integrate and maintain the wisdom received during coaching sessions. Death doula training adds another layer of support for her clients and their families.

When Diane isn't caregiving, she enjoys spending time in nature, learning new things, swing dancing—and being with her granddaughter!

If you are ready to:

- Reduce your stress from caregiving demands
- Prioritize yourself and enhance your well-being
- Expand your sense of purpose
- Heal emotionally, mentally, physically, and spiritually
- Shift to a positive mindset and
- Lay the groundwork for your vibrant future

Diane is here to guide and support you!

Connect with her at:

Website: https://www.dianemariegallant.com

Email: diane@dianemariegallant.com

Book: https://dianemariegallant.com/the-caregivers-advocate-finding-the-gift/

Facebook: https://www.facebook.com/dianemariegallant/

Instagram: https://www.instagram.com/diane_marie_gallant

LinkedIn: https://www.linkedin.com/in/diane-marie-gallant-6b1a083a/

CHAPTER 15

Stop the World; I Want to Get Off!

HOW TO STAY SANE WHILE CARING FOR YOUR LOVED ONE

R. Scott Holmes

THE STORY

Ugh, 3:30 a.m.!

Lying in the torture chamber rollaway cot, starving, scared, lost, humbled, and searching for anything to hold me together. I scuffed my way half-dressed to the communal bathroom, braving the spotlight and the echoes.

God, please let my little girl live. She is in the scariest place I have ever been: the Pediatric ICU. Please, let me take her place! Let me be the one stricken! Life would be so much easier if she didn't have to suffer. Please, it is in your hands.

In those twilight hours, I didn't understand the journey I had asked for.

Growing up in a middle-class neighborhood two blocks from each other, Moira and I knew all the same people, went to the same schools, and even worked on the same plays in high school, but we didn't meet until after graduation. Affection turned into love and transitioned into marriage: one daughter, two daughters, three daughters in six years. I worked two jobs so Moira could stay home and raise our growing family. Life was full of laughter, family, holidays, joys, and the dreams we had imagined.

Then, the terrifying call to work, Moira whimpered, "Something is wrong with Amanda. She woke up from her nap, and she won't respond."

Our daughter is in a zombie-like state.

Our lives changed forever.

Being 15 months old and the youngest meant she was the most energetic and engaging of our three daughters. But my wife could not get her to respond to any stimuli. "Meet me at the pediatrician's office. I'm calling right now."

Ten minutes away, I flew to the office. Walking into the overflowing waiting room, I walked over to where Moira was cradling Amanda. There was a slight twitch in the corner of Amanda's mouth. I immediately picked her up and led Moira to the doctor.

"She's starting to seize!"

Within five minutes, both on-duty doctors and a nurse were doing what they could to calm down a grand mal seizure in a child with no symptoms or history of any disorder. "We are sending her to Floating Hospital in Boston," Dr. Hourigan said. I looked at Moira's wide, fear-filled eyes, and we knew our little girl was in real trouble.

The ambulance inching through Boston rush hour, followed by hours of waiting and the not-knowing all seemingly endless torture.

The first time hearing our perfectly happy, healthy daughter cry, truly cry, was devastating.

Two days later, as we finally left the hospital, Amanda was in the Pediatric ICU with a bolt in her head to measure cranial pressure, an A-line in her thigh, and not much hope that she would survive the week as she was diagnosed with Herpes Encephalitis Simplex 2. A virus that devastates and destroys the brain. It stopped just short of killing her and left her in a coma.

Going home was the most important thing we had to do that day, as my two other daughters had not only lost their sister but their parents as well. We needed to reassure them we were okay and that however scared we might be, they would be alright.

Three months later, Amanda was transferred to our local hospital. Two weeks later, we had our comatose daughter at home. We were scared out of our minds but determined to give her the best chance of survival and the best quality of life.

For long-term caregivers—this story may sound familiar. Starting the journey and the emotional heartbreak was devastating because it was our child, our baby.

Now, for the rest of the story.

Quality of Life: Our five-room apartment housed Amanda's wheelchair, bean bag, overnight feeding pump, various medical supplies, and all we needed for caregiving. Everything was stacked, shoved, and shelved around our daily lives. The living room turned into the treatment room, where OT, PT, nurses, and aids came to help in a whirlwind of daily activity.

My other daughters were six and four years old, and Amanda's care became the normal daily routine, withholding from them the dreams of an ordinary childhood. Compounded by doctor's visits scheduled and unscheduled, activities canceled and changed depending on Amanda's well-being and living under the shadow of a sister whose care was life-consuming.

What is a 'normal' life when living in a volatile roller-coaster existence?

How do you determine what is best? For everyone?

Isolation: Although our families lived close, there was truly little time for social activity and connection. We endured the uncertainties, never knowing if we would be in a local hospital or Boston or how the day was going with Amanda. Each day was like being on a thrill ride for the first time, never knowing the twists and turns that were coming.

Every invitation was with the proviso, "If Amanda is okay." Shifting attendant schedules made for little time for extended family. Friends that in the past might call soon drifted away as the pressures of daily care and exhaustion crept in.

It was deeply isolating and lonely–between Moira and I and our daughters.

How can you seek connection and relief when it is your role and duty to provide minute-by-minute care and support for your child?

Money: I was working full time and Moira's full-time job was Amanda and the girls. As we were accepted for Social Security for Amanda, we were eligible for more help, but we were limited in how much money we could earn. I couldn't accept raises at work, an opportunity for a house was dashed, and sometimes deciding what to pay and when to pay became agonizing. Pressure grew each month as we got further behind in debt.

Our landlords worked with us. Family helped when and where they could. We told each other we would make this work.

Somehow. In some way, we did.

How do you balance all the limitations and feelings as if it's enough?

Grief: At the time, we mourned not only the loss of who Amanda was but also the potential of who she would have become. Our dreams of what life would be with three happy, healthy girls had vanished. So, too, had our life we had worked towards.

Moreover, Moira and I never got the chance to express our feelings or comfort each other through this ordeal, as life continuously kept throwing us more curveballs.

How do you grieve and comfort your beloved partner?

How do you heal the wounds when you are struggling to survive?

When there is barely life as it is right now?

Stress: Neither of us slept more than a couple of hours straight without waking to crying. Looking back, I do not know how we functioned. I was on autopilot, up early after a fitful sleep, and then I went to work. Moira was dog tired from the wear and care of each day. We never knew what the next day would bring and were always on high alert.

We were not as much husband and wife as we were partners in care. We took turns with breaks, which often meant shifting focus to our other two girls. As much help as we had coming into the house for Amanda, there was never a real respite for us.

How do you parent healthy daughters when the caregiving demands are so great?

Relationship: There is no one else in this world I would have gone side-by-side into battle with than Moira. 'For better or worse' never came up as we struggled to survive and create a family life. We were in this together and did whatever it took to see this journey through.

Moira was my partner, a fierce Momma Bear who was strong beyond measure and had the biggest, caring heart. Yet what love we had was poured into our children.

Fully.

Gratefully.

Exhaustively.

Leaving our relationship to weather the endless storms. The young love we felt early on was replaced with steeled determination.

Our definition of love changed. Our relationship deepened.

And sometimes, the divide seemed to expand as we navigated loneliness and aloneness.

How do you maintain a healthy, loving relationship?

When you have no energy left, your emotions are on edge, and you're waiting for the next piece of your life to crumble, how do you express your love?

Fear: Those closet monsters came out at 3 a.m. and filled the room as I stared wide-eyed, the little boy inside wanting to hide his head under the covers and pretend they didn't exist. Each monster tried to convince me, taunting me with my insecurities:

You are not able to provide.

You are losing those most precious things.

You are not up to the task.

You are not enough.

When those fears overtake you, how do you respond?

How are you able to shut those thoughts off in your mind?

As a parent, how do you deal with the feeling of failing to provide and protect your child?

Navigating the healthcare system: Every caregiver has enduring stories of healthcare failing their child. It is evident with a multiply impaired child how you are your child's advocate. When you're dealing with multiple agencies, hospitals, modalities, and insurance companies you must be that strong, rapidly learning, and knowing expert.

Amanda's three and a half months in Floating Hospital in Pediatric ICU, Intermediate Care, and then on a regular hospital floor cost over $250k in 1983 dollars, about $780k in 2024.

We shook every branch, spoke with so many agencies, talked with other parents, dealt with early intervention, state agencies, local hospitals, pediatricians, specialists, surgeons, neurologists, occupational and physical therapists, nurse practitioners, non-profit agencies, Boston hospitals, and insurance carriers.

Overwhelming? You betcha!

How can you find help and answers to the questions in the labyrinth that is health care?

Who can you trust to give you the right options to make the best decisions?

I could relate to numerous stories, anecdotes, graveyard humor, and mistakes made while caring for our daughters. The hardest and one that tested us the most was when we made a life-altering decision.

Massachusetts was only one of two states in the country that had pediatric nursing home beds. There were 260 beds in four nursing homes dedicated to the care and education of multiply impaired children until the age of 22. When we were first approached at Boston Floating Hospital to institutionalize our daughter, the thought was not even considered. Even though she was in a "comatose" state, we felt there was more that could be done.

So, we opted, after much consideration, to give Amanda every chance to have the best quality of life by bringing her home. After two and a half years of 24-hour care, we saw what the future would look like. We had brought Amanda to the point of recovery we could and had to consider what was best for her care and what our other daughters needed.

Our case manager arranged for us to submit the request and a board of 15 state employees would hear her acceptance for a bed. Moira and

I went to the hearing and, in a very unusual proceeding, allowed Moira and I to speak.

Questions from numerous departments were asked, and Moira answered them unwaveringly. Poker faces are all I saw as the hour rolled by. When asked if I wanted to add anything, I wanted to allow them to feel some of what we were feeling.

If my wife and I could continue to care for our daughter, we would do so. There is not enough help to care for Amanda and sustain any quality of life for her or our family. You may see this as giving us a placement, but we see it as giving up our daughter. Of letting her go. Of failing as a parent. You'll make your recommendations as you will; just know we have given all we have.

She was admitted into the Pediatric Nursing Home 40 minutes away. This was the start of our next hill to climb. Another institution, more personalities, new doctors, and other battles to ensure she had the best quality of life. In retrospect, it was a wonderful outcome for Amanda. For 12 years, she got quality 24-hour care, we got sleep and rest, and my daughters could enjoy school and growing up being big sisters to Amanda.

The phone ringing at 2 a.m. is never good.

"Mr. Holmes, I don't know any other way to say this, but Amanda has passed."

Dozens of times, we had rushed to the hospital expecting the worst after getting a call from the pediatric nursing home that took care of her. Without fanfare, an ambulance ride, or medics working on her as they had so many times before, Amanda had stopped breathing quietly in the middle of the night with no warning.

We spent 14 years on the roller coaster ride until she passed at 15 years old.

Our decisions and lessons learned as caregivers allowed us to appreciate life in all its fractured colors. If asked at the beginning of this journey, "Can you survive this?" I would have answered a firm NO!

Asked now? I wouldn't change a thing.

THE STRATEGY

In our journey, Moira and I educated medical staff and doctors about parents' rights. This was never more evident than when we were at a Boston hospital, sitting across from the world-famous head of the neurology department. An older doctor, he was used to respect and never being questioned. He was describing the treatment used for "children like this." My wife stood up from her chair, placed her hands on the desk, looked him straight in the eye, and said, "You work for us. We will determine what is and is not done with our daughter. I am her mother, and I have the last word." The ultimate rule follower became the ultimate Momma Bear.

Quality of Life: The filter we used when making any medical decision was what would give Amanda and our family the best quality of life. What results in the best for all? These are some of the hardest decisions we ever had to make.

Isolation: Parent support groups: in-person or virtual, respite care, accepting when friends and family ask for help, allowing friends to visit even though the house is in shambles. Federation for Children with Special Needs, https://fcsn.org is an organization geared for advocacy and support.

Money: When winning the lottery isn't enough, state and federal agencies listed in this book deliver in-kind services to local agencies. One such agency is Connect and Thrive, Inc., which lists where to find discounted and complimentary services.

Stress: There are agencies that'll give in-kind therapeutic services such as Reiki, massage, and respite care so you can relieve the tension. Allow yourself space and time wherever you can find it. It is self-care, not selfish.

Marriage: Statistics show that 75% of marriages with multiply impaired children end in divorce or separation. Communication, honesty, and trust are paramount to keeping the family together. Have the hard conversations before they are present in your relationship.

Fear: If you have ten minutes in a day, you can meditate. It takes many forms and can help minimize the fear monsters: online, quiet meditation, repeated mantras, walking in nature, and yoga. Find the one that fits.

Navigating the health care system: Learn to speak MEDICALESE. Learning the language spoken by your medical team ensures you can translate your child's story to medical professionals. They'll understand more clearly. You'll be heard. Finding a healthcare advocate through your state agencies will help guide you through the intricacies of modern medicine.

These are but a few suggestions as you maneuver through your child's journey. Know that you are not alone in experiencing the overwhelm and confusion. Reach out, find that trusted source, and know you will indeed make it through.

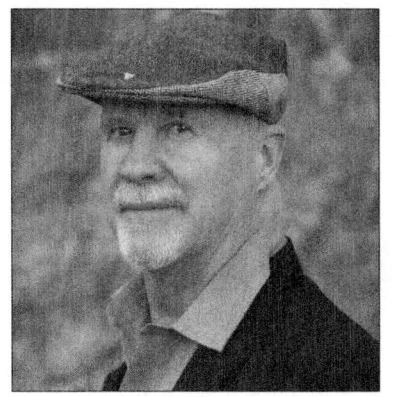

R. Scott Holmes is an intuitive energy practitioner and transformational coach using Reiki, polarity therapy, RYSE, ThetaHealing, and Find Your Voice coaching techniques to clear, ground, and align your energetic body. His specialty is collaborating with professional men and women, allowing them to heal and maintain their true paths in life.

He began walking in the holistic healing world when his wife of 39 years died after a 20-year battle with breast cancer. After years of caregiving for his daughter and wife, the world of coaching, healing, and energy opened. His soul journey has been to help heal others through one-on-one sessions, teaching, and volunteering.

Scott lives in Massachusetts and is delighted to share his spiritual journey, using his experiences to help heal and guide. Travel to Vietnam, Malaysia, India, Europe, and the UK has been a passion. Understanding people no matter where and how they live on this beautiful planet has become his *raison d'etre*. Seeing clients transform, grow, heal, awaken, and embrace why they were put on this planet is the ultimate reward for all who do this work.

Feeling overwhelmed? We can find your happy place.

Braving isolation? Learning solitude on this journey.

Not being heard? You can find your true voice.

Message or email Scott for a free half hour introduction session.

Website: https//www.rscottholmes.com
Contact him at rscott_holmes@yahoo.com
Facebook: https//www.facebook.com/Scott.Holmes.31105674
Instagram: https//www.instagram.com/r.scottholmes

CHAPTER 16

A Journey Through My Mother's Dementia

HOW TO NAVIGATE THE FOG OF GUARDIANSHIP

Frank Byrum

MY STORY

Tears streaming down her flushed cheeks, the little girl sniffled, "But it's time to plant my garden."

With my performance accomplished, I could finally breathe. *It's finished.*

There are no words, no wisdom, no saint that can assuage the anguish of saying, "Mom. You have dementia."

I must admit, I played along. All her children played along, letting her believe she would one day return home and plant her vegetable garden. At every request, my heart sank as I dodged the difficult questions and evaded interrogation.

Mom, you can't go home! You can never go home.

Each visit, I held my tongue until the hostilities grew, and then I retreated to the lonely drive home.

We agreed to tell her about this as a family, and with the doctors flanking—a pale green assisted-care room, clean, smelling of bleach. Locked in time, maybe from the 1950s, fitting the irony of dementia.

Her voice now at a boiling tone, reminiscent of my childhood discipline, with a flush hot crimson face.

She contended, "... but I have to do my paperwork!"

Oh yes, the paperwork.

For years, Mom talked about the paperwork. After decades as a schoolteacher, her paperwork was as common as fresh or canned garden veggies at dinner.

Years past retirement, I figured paperwork was bill paying, farm accounting, or related activities.

Little did I or anyone in the family understand that paperwork was her short-term memory.

I'm still perplexed about how she adjusted to a declining short-term memory— her paperwork (tens of small notepads). Writing notes is an obvious solution, but no one knew that her daily memories, observations, and thoughts were kept on small pads. Notes like:

Floyd, fresh croakers. (Mom fried many fish and hush puppies for her friends.)

Strange car. (Perhaps an unexpected or recognized visitor next door.)

Brenda called. (My sisters often called to check in.)

Inestimable scribbles throughout her day, and she learned to review them often. And so, she read her daily paperwork to each offspring, evidently repeating the same notes to each.

How brilliant. How amazing. How sad.

I didn't see how quickly Mom declined after Dad passed, or maybe she had already declined. Amid the creeping fog of dementia, her decline emerged with stark clarity, like the vividness of a sapphire sky obscured gradually by the rolling mists of an autumn morning, revealing a serene yet profound transformation.

She escalates—bawling. "I don't understand. There is nothing wrong with my memory!"

A friend taught me that two opposite things can be true. Mom's long-term memory and recollection were truly remarkable—detailed family trees, a daughter of the soil—picking tomatoes and truck crops, recounting friends, holidays, and vacations.

And her students, seemingly by the hundreds, recognized her. They all remembered the smells of slightly sweet, yeasty dinner rolls or caramelized brown sugar and chocolate chip cookies of home economics class.

Mom's paperwork was convincing until it wasn't.

Between Dad's retirement and her school pension, Mom was well-fixed. After multiple petitions, "Frank, can you help me pay for Christmas dinner this year?"

"Of course, Mom, anything you need?"

Later Mom was "a little short" for bills.

I kept telling myself, *something is awry*.

A neighbor, a scumbag, a rapscallion, 30 years her junior; her "love." He and his mother were regular dinner guests. Nearing 80—her mind rapidly depreciating, along with her accounts.

His recompense was harmless at first, as was the payment for painting a room and a few home repairs. This interloper convinced my infirmed mother they could start a restaurant together. It was only later he impersonated me, her only son, to sign for a reverse mortgage on her house.

His daring ruse was exposed when she became sick and had to enter assisted living.

I can't recall her words after the paperwork plea—firing mad, I've hidden the hurtful words from myself. There are two things true about Mom: 1) she was an amazingly generous and sweet person, and 2) at times, she was a force and tempest that I learned to avoid as a small child.

Since I was the bad news messenger, I silently dismissed myself and let my sisters and others finish up. It seemed I was always delivering the bad news, and it was clear that even though she couldn't remember why, she was nervous when I dropped by with everyone.

In retrospect, it was all clear.

At first, it's the chair that helped her stand after kneeling. Then she entered the room without remembering why. Then, it was the conversation that didn't exactly make sense, and after a few questions, she could talk her way out of the conundrum. She's likely reading her paperwork.

Now, in my 60s, all this seems normal.

If we live long enough, we'll age and grow frail.

And so, her memory fog was on little notepads; these were everywhere—by the bed, her reading chair, in her pocketbooks, her dresser, on the counter, in her housecoat—the clouds of her memory strewn all over the house.

On the slow walk to my car, I remember myself as a small boy hugging Mom in her rocking chair as she hummed to comfort me while my little hand patted her back, "Mom, I will take care of you."

There was nothing I could do to take care of her now. Even my science and engineering skills were of no use.

The next morning, I sat in my daily practice, trying to recall the fog, now a blur that led up to everything.

The hundreds of small discrepancies—the first inkling she might have a problem. Ultimately leading to the doctor baselining her mental decline, a key piece of evidence for what became guardianship.

My own fog was interrupted. *Why did my 4-year-old self say I would take care of her? What preceded that statement? What was going on with Mom that day?* Her tears are etched into my memory as I sought to comfort her. Now, I marvel at how a boy could grasp the depth of such unhappiness.

One look back as I left the solemn moment, Mom had slumped into a lump, silently weeping. The youngest of my three sisters, kneeling at her side, patting her hand. The little boy had failed—*I had failed.*

Months before, the lawyer was clear, "It's not so easy to reverse guardianship, and it was a big responsibility." Sadly, none of her children were able to provide around-the-clock care. Dementia was an evil spirit, an endless fog, keeping her up at all hours—angry and confused.

A suitable guardian agency was assigned—in our area, Jewish Services or Catholic Services. Both had stellar reputations, and Jewish Services supported our family and performed an amazing job while we focused on visiting and loving her through her last years.

The months turned into years, and as she declined, she required the next level of care. Until she was in a lockdown ward with an ankle security tracking bracelet and finally a wheelchair.

It was hard to visit her. She wasn't my mom, although she bore a striking resemblance, especially in her now azure eyes, which had turned from her natural chatoyant hazel due to dementia. The first year or so, each visit was short. The pleading was the same, "Please let me go home to my garden," she cried, and the initial fog turned into a nasty tempest.

And then, one day, she wasn't. As time passed, the storm became a settled fog. Mom became a sweet little old lady who liked me to visit but couldn't recall my name. However, I received a big smile, bright eyes, and many old memories on each visit, especially about her garden and family.

At one low point, she said, "Lewis came by and. . . (I couldn't make out her words) we're going and. . . it rained. . ." And then the biggest smile and laughter I had ever seen.

It was contagious. I laughed, too, and then I cried.

From then on, I didn't understand much she said. However, if I caught a word now and then, I'd make up a related question. When she was in her silent haze, I was just asking her about her garden or growing up; I rarely understood anything. However, she grinned and giggled after each story, which always pierced my gloom. We laughed a lot, and I don't really know why. But it seemed to please her. Every drive home, the tears flowed. We needed to resolve so much, and those days had passed.

In her failing days, she was nearly a skeleton. She had lost so much weight, refusing to eat. My sister closest in age and I sat with her the night before she passed. I patted her hand, still haunted by, *Mom, I will take care of you.* The little boy, now the grown man, is trying to do the impossible.

It was no more possible for me to clear her mental fog as that innocent little boy patting her back.

In the end, the guardianship truly helped our family. We could focus on being present when visiting—that was hard enough—and working to settle her house and lifetime of accumulations.

Looking back, I've come to believe in sainthood, especially for those who care for dementia patients. Or maybe they are just the children of angels.

Today, I'm reminded that if I live long enough, maybe I, too, will decline. I may live in a fog, and my loved ones may struggle to navigate the uncertainty.

If coping with Mom's mental fog wasn't hard enough, guardianship was even murkier. We asked her doctor to give her a mental test—Mini-Mental Status Examination (MMSE). There are several possible tests. However, each is designed to check mental abilities. This was a critical step because it serves as a baseline for future evaluations. In my experience, there were days when Mom seemed credibly okay, and, in the early days, it was difficult to detect.

On reflection, I can see she was guarded and often avoided detailed short-term memory discussions. Oddly, she kept her small pad next to her dinner plate.

The legal fogbank was even denser to penetrate. Elder law is a specialty. We quickly realized she was being exploited, which complicated things. The line between gifts and exploitation is difficult to prove and resolve before guardianship can be awarded.

Persistence pays off. While it's bothersome, you must work through the daily drizzle and haze, part by part, until you have reached clarity. A few considerations on guardianship:

- Guardianship is a brave act by a family for a loved one who is no longer capable of making informed decisions due to their condition.
- Guardians will help a loved one unable to secure the appropriate medical care, manage their medication, or make decisions. This can lead to untreated medical conditions, accidents, or exposure to abuse and exploitation.
- Guardians may help avert financial abuse, fraud, or exploitation. Especially over financial transition and they may be easy prey for

financial scams and may lose their financial security, leading to debt or even homelessness.

- Guardians will protect against manipulation or unauthorized legal decision, contracts, or legal agreements, and offer guidance for individuals when considering legally binding decisions, such as living arrangements.
- Guardians may help families navigate disagreements in care, finances, and medical treatments.
- Guardians will help navigate the complex legal and bureaucratic healthcare, social services, and financial aid.

Guardianship is a difficult step, and I admit it wasn't an easy decision for my family and me. It was time-consuming, and we were late in helping our mother. She was exploited and lost a significant amount of money.

It's important to set aside time for you as an individual and as a family to discuss this difficult matter. Realize your loved one may not understand their need and may not cooperate. For those families, my prayers and hopes are with you on your journey.

For me, the spiritual practices I embraced decades past stand as a beacon in the gloominess, granting me the grace to peer through the mist of yesteryears, to ponder our collective choices, and to navigate my healing path daily with newfound clarity.

THE STRATEGY

Select a quiet place and give yourself time: I recommend having no activities planned for at least 30 minutes longer than your planned meditation length to avoid feeling rushed. When initially starting, it's important not to be emotionally rushed by your next activity.

In my practice, I brew a small pot of tea, bring a pen and writing pad, and sit outside, away from distractions.

The secret is the tea or coffee is a cue; over time, it will become an internal reminder to your soul that you are about to enter your practice. Throughout the day, the same cue enables you to practice a mindful pause, relax, and breathe for a few minutes with a late morning or afternoon cup.

Brain chatter is normal, so don't fret, don't resist, and embrace the chatter: today's to-do list, meetings, memories, anger, anything. Give yourself permission to attend to these later and write each on the pad as they appear.

Note: replace your loved one's name where I underlined <u>her pronoun</u>. Consider a few prayerful thoughts:

How is <u>her</u> health, and is she capable of taking care of herself?

Do I recognize struggles in <u>her</u> ability to take care of herself?

How would I describe <u>her</u> decision-making ability?

Does <u>she</u> seem to be having issues?

Has <u>her</u> doctor performed a mental acuity test yet?

Additional Steps:

- Understand how to recognize the signs of dementia.
- Discuss your observations with her doctor and request a baseline evaluation.
- Consult with an elder law attorney to understand your jurisdiction requirements. Your attorney will help with the petition of guardianship, which includes associated evidence and terms.
- Document, document, document. Collect your observation and a copy of all medical, financial, and legal documents.
- Consider interviewing professional guardian organizations in your area. Specifically, request or pay close attention to reviews.
- Check in with the guardian and ensure they provide appropriate court filings, including health and financial statuses.
- Visit. The best evidence is in seeing the care for yourself. While it may be emotionally hard, do not neglect your loved one.

This may seem gratuitous to imply—take care of yourself. A wise friend taught me, "The leaning fence post falls first." If you are going through this process or visiting your loved one during their declining years, it is deeply emotional, stressful, and, often, guilt-ridden. Realize that your best is what you can do today.

Don't neglect your daily practice. Please see my website for ideas and resources.

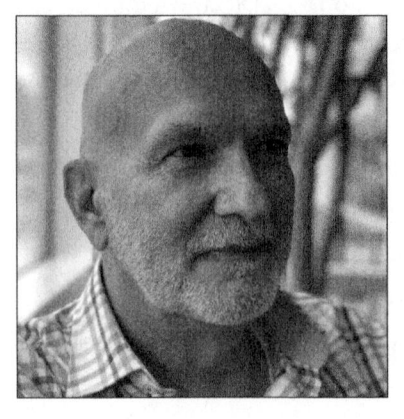

Frank Byrum is an inventor & scientist, technologist, and best-selling author who has spent the last four decades on a spiritual journey, the last few of which have focused on deep self-healing. His dad led his early spiritual training in the Southern Baptist tradition; following in his footsteps, he continued the family tradition as a Bible teacher for several decades.

To continue his religious education, he began a Master of Theology in Apologetics, and it was during this time that he began to consider the teachings deeply and realized few taught or even mimicked Jesus' love, kindness, and healing. Ultimately, not completing the degree and with this soul-belief—what was once known and practiced has been lost.

This questioning, this crisis of faith, led to decades of searching various wisdom traditions and teachers, and with a simple faith believing the promise of Mathew 7:7— "Ask, and it shall be given you; seek, and ye shall find; knock, and it shall be opened unto you" (KJV).

For years, he's shared his understanding with friends, family, students, and associates as he continued researching and practicing. He earnestly believes everyone can benefit from the foundation of a practical daily practice, and it's the best way to "be in the world, but not of the world." Today, his daily practice includes tea, breath work, prayer and meditation, martial arts katas, Qi-Gong energy work, and wisdom studies. He resides in southern Virginia, where he practices, teaches, and writes.

Download a PDF of the exercise and a guided audio:
https://themindfulpathway.com
Connect with Frank:
Website: themindfulpathway.com
Email: frank@themindfulpathway.com
Twitter: https://twitter.com/MindfulPathway or @MindfulPathway
Instagram: https://www.instagram.com/tfbyrum

CHAPTER 17

Alzheimer's and Rehabilitation

COULD AN INTEGRATIVE APPROACH BE THE ANSWER?

Nicky Sargant, Alzheimer's Live-in Carer

MY STORY

MEETING ANN

Everyone had left. All had gone well with Ann until I started cooking. Suddenly, I felt panic's piercing grip grab hold of me: weakness in my knees, my sickening heart tumbled to the pit of my stomach on hearing for the tenth time in three minutes, a lamented utter,

"It's awful, it's awful!"

Turning from the stove, I froze as I watched Ann standing by the counter, wrenching her hands in a highly agitated manner.

Oh God, please help me! I'm going to go mad.

What am I going to do? It'll be a long two weeks.

That split second seemed like an eternity of hellish anguish. All I could do was helplessly stand there. This was the first time I had cared for someone with Alzheimer's.

Now what?

Then reason kicked in. I knew it wasn't about me. My thoughts were racing.

This poor lady is afraid.

Who am I, someone new once again?

I need to comfort and help her to feel safe. I need to do it now!

I immediately removed the pan from the stove and walked over to her, stood by her side, and gently cradled her hands in mine. Slowly, her hands relaxed. She turned to me and smiled.

My heart welled up with relief, "Ann, are you okay?"

Her smile broadened. I offered her a cup of tea. She nodded, and while still holding her hand, we prepared the tea and found choccy biscuits to dip into it.

I watched with intrigue the sheer enjoyment on Ann's face as she bit into her biscuit, melting away the earlier heart-breaking scenes from my mind. Seeing Ann more relaxed, I leaned forward and made small talk with her. The outgoing carer had warned me Ann only spoke four words: yes, no, and thank you. In that moment, I realized the need to dig deep, think outside the box, and find ways to connect with Ann so her inability to communicate verbally wouldn't be a hindrance.

How can I possibly manage that? Seems almost impossible, but I must at least try.

FINDING A WAY

I'm sure many of you can identify. Maybe a flashback comes to mind of a similar situation where you, too, were unsure, perhaps felt panicked, or out of your depth.

It's not a nice place to be. I felt inadequate; it aches seeing someone in distress when you can't reach or help them.

I decided in that moment I needed to read up on Alzheimer's and research as much as I could. There was such a gentleness about Ann that really pulled at my heartstrings. She deserved the very best I could give her.

Over the following days, I scoured the internet.

Oh no! It all sounds awful!

Finding nothing positive, my heart saddened. Everywhere I looked was doom and gloom.

A slow death sentence, in short, and often a very painful one.

In desperation, I searched for natural remedies, and a glimmer of hope appeared. One thing led to another. Food started showing up and its effects on Alzheimer's. Inflammation and antioxidants were quoted.

What's an antioxidant? Why is it so important?

Leaky gut! What's that?

Mitochondria?

A stomach-like ecosystem within us, with good and bad bacteria? That could lead to leaky brain?

Heavy metals, toxins, etc., entering the brain and destroying parts of it?

Seriously, this is sounding like a sci-fi horror movie!

Amongst all this terrible news, talk about how diet and lifestyle changes help heal the gut and brain surfaced. Looking at foods that create a healthy gut, I stumbled upon Dr. Axe.

Wow, this stuff is amazing!

Fats, oils, Mediterranean diets, spices, turmeric in particular, you name it, the list was endless, too many to mention. The more I delved in, the more I uncovered. Most of it was practical, simple, and doable!

Dr. Mary Newport, helping her husband using coconut oil?

The most amazing was a doctor in the US working on a protocol for Alzheimer's. He was definitely making waves in the medical fraternity. Although in early stages, it showed much promise.

The Bredesen Protocol? What's that all about? Could he be on to something?

It took me a while to get my head around this new information. I was skeptical at first, even dismissive. One link led to another and another. A sea of information was out there. My head exploded with uncertainty and disbelief. Slight panic began to emerge within.

So confusing and overwhelming!

The only thing I knew was the more I read, the more sense it made. Endless studies have been conducted by so many different doctors who crossed the floor in favor of this new medicine.

Looking for the root causes and treating them rather than treating the symptoms! What does that mean?

Why aren't we hearing more of this instead of all the negative and depressing information?

This was head-scratching stuff with too many such studies emerging. It was becoming very hard to ignore.

Organically grown and reared food versus pesticides and hormonal-induced food?

Chemicals and preservatives used in manufacturing and processing can ultimately poison the gut and brain?

As I leaned back in my chair, I thought,

Wow, all these things are so carefully and miraculously intertwined.

It's all beginning to fall into place.

I stared in amazement.

Could it be so simple?

In theory, yes, but practically, no!

Where are these experts?

What tests are required to determine in what stage or state the body is, that's affecting the brain?

I don't know any doctors who practice that.

During the remaining three years, I was honored to oversee and care for Ann. Orchestrated through family chats, changes were slowly introduced to improve Ann's quality of life and fill her with as much joy as possible.

Sugars were greatly reduced, and a gut-friendly diet together with coconut oil was introduced (after confirming with Ann's doctor on a daily spoonful).

LIVING JOYFULLY

We puttered around the garden, watering the flowerbeds with her hilarious little dance. Just as the conductor moves from one stringed instrument to the next, she moved the spray from one flower to the next with meticulous precision, serenading each one with a "chuu, chuu, chuu."

We went for long walks. Ann loved nature and the outdoors. She often pointed saying, "Look," upon seeing a pretty flower or the vapor trail of a plane in the clear blue sky.

We went out to places: shopping, coffee shops, visiting friends, etc. The more we did, the more engaging she became.

Music became a huge part of our lives, making it my favorite 'go-to' tool. Ann loved to dance! We literally danced our way through each day. Her eyes lit up every time we danced to either the radio or a CD. Ann loved all types of music, especially classical with her background in opera and ballet.

Later, after reading the amazing studies on classical music and how it lights up the brain and improves memory, I smiled. I was on the right track after all.

One of my fondest memories of Ann and music involved a day trip to London. We were in Peter Jones strolling through the radios and CD players, and then came the Bose headphones. I picked up a headset and placed it on Ann's head. She started listening, bopping away to the music. She was staring at the jack plugged into a board but couldn't see the player behind it. Surprise was written all over her face; *where's the music coming from?* Then an, *oh well*, she started bopping again. She turned to me and smiled, unknowingly dislodging the jack connection at the same time. Aghast, she turned back, wondering *what the heck happened?* I plugged it back in, and the cycle continued, her listening, accidentally unplugging it, and my plugging it back in. Each time it happened, the shock and disappointment on her face were priceless.

Ann became more and more relaxed, adventurous, and trusting as she connected with me and those around her. Smiling and laughing replaced her agitation and weeping. She started adding words to her vocabulary, even short sentences!

The most exciting was one day after our walk I asked her, "Do you fancy a cuppa?"

I nearly fell over when she casually replied, "That would be lovely."

CARING FOR MYSELF

As a carer, I'm constantly on high alert: looking, checking, and accessing for potential risks. This allows the person for whom I'm caring the freedom to be and do as much as possible. Carers know only too well how exhausting and draining caregiving is. It's incredibly easy to lose oneself in the person being cared for and their needs.

I remember a professional once pulling me up on it, saying, "You can't look after others if you don't look after yourself."

I had a real problem with that statement because that's what carers do. We care for others, whether we're carers, spouses, mothers, etc. Right? However, she was spot on! It just took me a while to see it. Now I get it. Do I still battle with self-care? Absolutely!

I do my best to take "stolen moments." It may be just a few minutes standing outside when safe to do so, sipping a cup of coffee.

Damn! That tastes good.

It's all about allowing yourself some headspace, and I have learned to be creative in this one!

When caregiving becomes too much, a walk with that person is a real lifesaver. There's something magical about being out in nature: fresh air on your face, blowing through your hair, the song of the birds, and greeting those you pass on the street. Moving into a calmer environment not only relaxes and re-energizes but transcends to you both. This little hack of walking or driving with music on (but not too loud of course) has saved my sanity a thousand times over.

Living in gratitude was another thing I learned to maintain my sanity. It's catchy! I remember reading a lot about this, initially thinking, *what a joke!* But I practiced it by writing down three things a day for which I was grateful. It took a while, but it began to help. Now, I know I can't do what I do unless I'm continually in a state of gratitude. I also have an amazing God, so I'm sorted!

A couple years into caring, I remember listening to a lady give a TED talk which had such an impact on me. She peered into the audience and said,

"I ask each of you to turn to the right and look at the person next to you."

What she stated next shook me to the core.

"Within your lifetime, one of you will either get dementia or be a carer for someone with dementia."

She was emphasizing the expected dementia increase. It made me stop and think seriously about my life and the risks I take daily as a carer.

Am I still a live-in carer? Yes! Am I still scared? Absolutely!

From what I have learned over the years, I do my best to maintain a healthy lifestyle. I know I need to listen to my body and be kind to myself so I can be there for others.

Caring can be lonely and isolating, as you're it! Taking time out at the end of the day to unwind before going to bed is imperative. It's beneficial to evaluate and top up for the next day.

Over the last eight years, I've been fortunate to cross paths with some amazing people doing incredible work and studies. Researchers have been pinpointing how an unhealthy lifestyle, sleep deprivation, lack of exercise, unhealthy foods, and a toxic environment can affect our modern-day life and the onset of Alzheimer's.

Time and time again, studies have proven enormous changes for the worse to our physical, mental, and emotional well-being today compared to years gone by. Stress, mental health issues, and new debilitating diseases are on the increase, too numerous to mention. These never existed in the past, but sadly are now affecting our young children and even babies.

It's impossible not to step back and gasp in horror.

Is there a connection?

We can choose to either accept or ignore it.

I'm fast learning the importance of taking charge of my health. This means being responsible and making informed decisions based on my newly found knowledge; weighing up all the options, choosing which path to follow, and what feels most comfortable.

If the day ever comes when I feel cognitively impaired, my visit will be to a doctor with a protocol to treat me based on my root causes, not my symptoms.

I'm often amazed at the times I've tweaked other's lifestyles for the better and witnessed positive changes by using a minuscule of information and knowledge that is out there.

Knowledge is power.

Our minds are sacred and need to be safeguarded. When we lose our minds, we lose our independence, and later our dignity. Then our life.

THE STRATEGY

'If only I knew then what I know now' can be haunting words.

Perhaps you are where I was and wondering where to begin.

The notes below outline some of the most important strategies I have learned. I hope they can be just as useful to you as they have been to me.

Step 1. The need to feel connected, loved, and valued

- Family members know the background of their loved ones, what lights them up, and what makes them tick.
- Paid carers have no clue. They can only work with what they see and learn along the way from either the person, their family, or their friends.

Tips:

- Compile a brief history: who the person was, what they did, what they were like.

- Learn their achievements, life's defining moments, hobbies, interests, likes, dislikes, and interesting facts about them.
- This knowledge allows carers a head start in fostering a connection into gaining the person's trust.

Step 2. Connection + Trust = The Magic Begins

- Caring is a journey traveled together.
- A care partnership is built on connection and trust, which transforms into a beautiful, fun, and rewarding relationship.
- It takes time, lots of time!

Tips:

- Hanging out is greatly beneficial and enriching for both.
- Knowing the history allows the carer to recreate activities once enjoyed by adapting them to suit the current capabilities.

Step 3. Patience, Compassion, and Empathy

- Alzheimer's changes the functionality and cognitive behavior of a person, but the person within is still the same, still existing. It's easy to lose sight of this.
- Understanding the person is vital to serving them.
- Often, when the person acts out, it's a silent cry for feeling trapped, unable to connect, frightened, or isolated.
- It's not their fault that they are unable to connect with you. It's the disease.
- The way you connected before the diagnosis may be lost. Learn to adapt and find new ways of connecting.
- It's a process of continual adaption.

"Mom doesn't want to get up. I'm tired of dragging her out of bed. I give up!"

No, it's not always stubbornness.

- Bed is her safe space.
- She can't be picked on for no longer understanding, being too slow, or battling to do simple tasks.

- She may be feeling unwanted and unloved. She may be feeling like a nuisance, a burden, or even fearful and ashamed of who she has become.

Tips:
- Put yourself in her shoes and remember it's not about you.
- Work *with* her, not *against* her; then life will flow with ease.
- Never underestimate what she feels, senses, or experiences.
- She's more intuitive than you realize.
- Reach out. Rescue her, in love.

Step 4. Diet
- The US Food Pyramid features bread, pasta, cereal, and rice as the major foods to consume at its base.
- Fats, oils, and sweets are at the top, and we are warned to eat less of them.

In the words of Dr. Dale Bredesen, "It turns out that this is a good recipe for giving ourselves obesity, insulin resistance, diabetes, hypertension, and cognitive decline - exactly what so many of us suffer from."

Tips:
- Nowadays, thanks to functional medicine, we have a clearer understanding of how the body is affected by the food we consume.
- The Brain Food Pyramid puts cognition-enhancing foods and practices such as fasting, healthy fats, and non-starchy vegetables on the base.
- Processed food, wheat, and dairy (due to intolerances) are to be avoided.
- Eight glasses of water daily keep the body and brain well-hydrated.
- The above tips promote an anti-inflammatory diet.

Step 5. Exercise
- Doing some form of movement every day is vital.
- It helps prevent depression.

- It prevents further memory loss by stimulating the production of hormones and neurotransmitters for memory retention learning.
- It's a mood elevator.
- Exercise reduces restlessness, wandering, and jitteriness.
- It helps maintain mobility and coordination for as long as possible, reducing the risk of falls that cause common hip injuries.
- It helps support the survival of existing neurons and promotes new neuron growth in the brain.

Tips:
- Make exercise easy and fun.
- Walk daily.
- Dance like nobody's watching.
- Chair exercises are an excellent option for immobility.

Step 6. Sleep
- Lack of sleep causes further impaired cognition and memory, fatigue, irritability, fussiness, forgetfulness, depression, lack of motivation, and clumsiness.
- Sleep cleanses and washes the brain.
- Less than 7-8 hours a night causes brain fog the next morning.

Tips:
- Routinely going to bed early helps the body clock.
- Leave a night light on to lessen the risk of falling.
- A dark room can be scary, causing them to feel unsettled.
- Keep the room at a comfortable temperature.

My wish is that I have sparked some intrigue within you to explore an integrative approach as I have described. Wherever you may be on this journey, I encourage you to hold on to hope that you will see more of the person emerge as you follow these strategic steps.

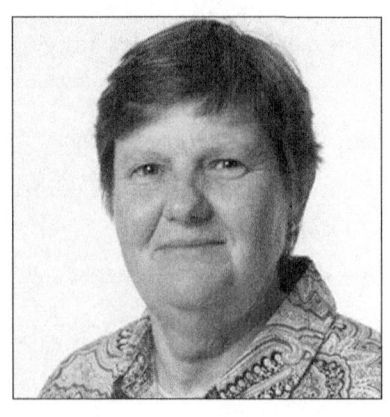

Nicky Sargant is an Alzheimer's Advocate, Ambassador, and Champion. Her primary goal is to create awareness by promoting a change of mindset in the ways people with Alzheimer's are managed, cared for, and treated. She has eight years of experience as a 24/7 live-in carer for the elderly, predominately those diagnosed with Alzheimer's. She has journeyed alongside them and witnessed their struggles. Many of the challenges have been painful and degrading for her clients. Some have faced discrimination, particularly medical, simply because they were unable to verbally communicate their pains, desires, or needs. In one particular case, her voice advocated for changes involving increased dementia-friendly care in a hospital setting.

Sargant's modern integrative approach to caring centers around lifestyle and the positive and negative effects on the delicately interconnected relationship between the gut and brain. She encourages a lifestyle of healthy diet, sleep, and exercise, along with music and stimulation, to prevent the onset of dementia and to maintain the highest quality of life for those who are already living with Alzheimer's.

Her mission is to spread awareness of the dangers and risk factors occurring from irresponsible farming and animal husbandry methods. She also raises awareness of the effects of ultra-processed foods on the gut, brain, and body.

Sargant is in the process of writing a book called *An Alzheimer's Journey of Hope: A Modern Approach to Caring*. Based on her personal carer experiences, the book will focus on a modern concept of managing and caring for people who have Alzheimer's. A 2024 release date is projected.

When not caring, Sargant loves to travel. Her penultimate is watching the sunset over the beach on a hot summer's eve, sipping a beer shandy surrounded by her adventurous, fun-loving nephews.

Connect with Nicky

LinkedIn: https://www.linkedin.com/in/nicky-sargant?trk=contact-info

CHAPTER 18

Love's Resilience and Hope

NAVIGATING MARRIAGE AFTER STROKE AND APHASIA

Michelle Briggs,
Spouse and Psychiatric Mental Health Nurse Practitioner

MY STORY

It was a beautiful day on April 11th, 2015. I was driving my sons, a friend, and my mother to the Eastern Shore for a fun weekend on the beach. John, my husband of a mere year and a half, was returning from a trip to Florida. He had been visiting his friends for several weeks, and the plan was to meet at our home in a few days. Excitedly, I called to tell him we had arrived. No answer. I unpacked for a while and tried again. No answer. *Hmm.* I opened up the app "Life 360," and the location of his phone was at a hospital. Instinct took over—my heart raced, pounding, and my head spun.

I called the emergency room. "Hello, this is John Bahel's wife. Does he happen to be there?" I waited, and the doctor answered the phone and confirmed that John was there. He asked about his medications and then told me they needed to do a procedure to break up a clot in his brain.

"Your husband could die without this procedure."

"Yes, yes, do it."

The procedure was completed, and John was on his way to shock trauma after suffering a left middle cerebral artery stroke. Without warning, our marriage would never be the same. My husband, best friend, and stepfather to my sons needed me to make life and death decisions for him, and it was time for us to navigate uncharted waters together. Could we withstand and overcome this challenge? Did we have the capacity to adapt, bounce back, and grow stronger together in the face of this adversity?

The "stroke" took on a life of its own. That day, it stole John's independence, speech, mobility, memory, emotional regulation, and strength. It took his dignity and fortitude. He became dependent on me to manage his life, and I was thrust into the role of caregiver wife. We had built a foundation of love and resilience in our marriage, yet it was crumbling. There was a sudden shift in my responsibilities, and now I was in the role of guardian, advocate, therapist, and financial navigator.

Love in a marriage is a deep and complex emotion that forms the foundation of a solid and fulfilling partnership. It goes beyond the initial attraction and evolves into a deep connection, respect, and commitment between two individuals.

Resilience in a marriage requires effective communication, mutual support, trust, and a willingness to work through problems as a team. Building a resilient marriage takes time, effort, and commitment from both individuals involved.

A stroke can significantly impact the love and resilience of a marriage. We were suddenly on a physical, spiritual, emotional, and psychological roller-coaster ride. And John's type of stroke had another challenge to overcome that I will call "Mount Aphasia."

John's stroke resulted in a diagnosis of expressive and receptive aphasia. Aphasia is a communication disorder that affects a person's ability to understand and use language effectively. When someone experiences a stroke with aphasia, the resilience requirement of effective communication between husband and wife is extinguished. You immediately become a mind reader, and the question, "What would he say in this situation?" becomes your compass.

Here are some metaphors that can help illustrate the experience:

1. Locked in a silent room: Imagine being in a room where you can see and hear what's happening around you but cannot speak effectively. Your thoughts and emotions are trapped inside. Your partner desperately wants to enter the room with you but doesn't know the lock code, and you can't tell them.
2. Broken telephone line: Think of a telephone line with static or interruptions, making it difficult to have a clear conversation. Feel the frustration and emotional strain of wanting to be heard clearly and watching your partner cry because they can't understand what you're saying and can't meet your needs.
3. Lost in a fog: Picture yourself in a dense fog, where words become muffled and difficult to find. You're struggling, and your partner interrupts your process to help you find the words, yet you just can't.
4. Puzzle pieces missing: Imagine trying to complete a puzzle, but some pieces still need to be included, and some are missing. Neither of you can find the pieces, and you're gripped by frustration.
5. Foreign language: Consider the experience of being in a foreign country where you don't speak the language. Everything around you is unfamiliar, and you struggle to communicate and understand others. You're both at the mercy of interpreting body language for your answers.

Aphasia made it extremely difficult for John to express his thoughts, needs, and emotions effectively. He could only write his name. His "yes" was a "no," and his "no" was a "yes." Our marriage entered a land of frustration and misunderstandings. John's inability to communicate created a sense of isolation and disconnect. I had so many questions for him. I never knew what he was really thinking. We were no longer a team working through problems.

A stroke with aphasia also requires significant adjustments in the roles and responsibilities within a marriage. I managed hospitalizations, rehabilitation facilities, assisted living facilities, and eventually, a home agency and caregivers. I became John's voice. Surprisingly, the general medical and rehabilitation staff were not educated on how to help John or myself navigate the extra support needed for aphasia. We began to rely heavily on the speech therapy staff, who explained that John may never be able to communicate effectively again.

"Only time will tell, and everyone is different." They educated us and referred us to https://aphasia.org for support. Eventually, John joined The Snyder Center for Aphasia Life Enhancement (SCALE) Program, and we were given the specialized support we needed. The program provided a place to connect and offered in-person interactive group activities to support people of all ages with aphasia. John had always liked helping others, and the program allowed him to assist speech therapy students in learning how to help patients with aphasia. And he made some great friends along the way.

We navigated the stroke storm for 3,266 days. John passed away on March 20, 2024. I will never know his most profound and intimate thoughts about the last nine years because he never regained much of his language. However, we created a language we understood. The kind of language that is heartfelt, spoken with the eyes and gestures of love and sometimes the middle finger. No one goes into a marriage expecting something like this to happen. Yet, you do your best to make it suitable for the "we" you each created.

I've learned a lot about life and loss these past nine years. I will never know what John learned. Yet I must accept "life on life's terms" and see that hope continues to rise in me. I am grateful for John and the lessons the stroke journey taught. I learned I have the strength to walk with purpose throughout life's challenges. I was and will always be a loving witness to another's journey. Loving yourself is the golden key to loving others. John would agree.

THE STRATEGY

Coping with aphasia in a marriage requires patience, understanding, and support. Here are some strategies that can help:

1. Seek professional help: Speech therapy can help the affected partner improve communication skills. Couples therapy or counseling can also provide a supportive environment to address the emotional impact of aphasia on the marriage.

2. Learn alternative communication methods: Explore alternative forms of communication, such as using visual aids, gestures, or technology-based communication tools. These methods can help enhance and maintain a connection between partners.

3. Foster empathy and understanding: Strive to understand each other's experiences and perspectives. Breathe and try to actively listen, be patient, and find ways to support each other emotionally.

4. Maintain social connections: Encourage the affected partner to participate in social activities and support groups designed for individuals with aphasia. This can reduce social isolation and provide opportunities for shared experiences.

5. Take care of yourself: The unaffected partner will benefit significantly from self-care activities and seek support from friends, family, or support groups.

6. Explore new ways to intimacy: Intimacy is not solely dependent on verbal communication. Focus on nonverbal forms of intimacy, such as touch, eye contact, and body language. Try activities like cuddling or massage, or engage in activities that you both enjoy. These can be powerful ways to connect and express love.

7. Forgive yourself: Remind yourself that you didn't cause the stroke and its effects; you cannot change what happened, and you cannot control the outcomes. Holding onto guilt and shame will only prolong your suffering and the suffering of your partner.

8. Learn from your experience: Use the experience as an opportunity for growth. Ask yourself what lessons you can take away from the situation. This mindset can help you move forward.

And, when you are feeling impatient, and your heart is restless:

"Be patient toward all that is unsolved in your heart and try to love the questions themselves, like locked rooms and like books that are now written in a very foreign tongue. Do not now seek the answers which cannot be given you because you would not be able to live them. And the point is, to live everything. Live the questions now. Perhaps you will then gradually, without noticing it, live along some distant day into the answer."

~ Letters to a Young Poet, Rainer Maria Rilke

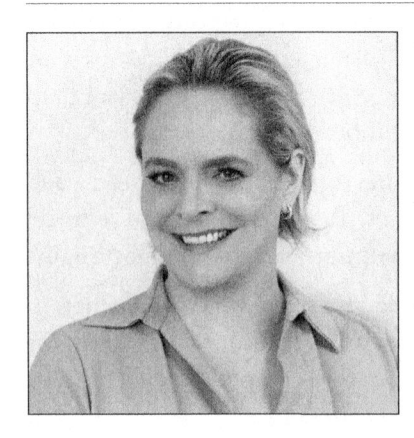

Michelle Briggs, a Psychiatric Mental Health Nurse Practitioner, owns Michelle Briggs, Integrative Psychiatry, and is the CEO of Code Green Healthcare, LLC, which specializes in cannabinoid therapeutics in Maryland. She has a Bachelor's of Nursing from Johns Hopkins University School of Nursing and a Master's of Nursing from the University of Maryland School of Nursing.

She spent 32 years in psychiatric nursing practice, and 6 of those have included recommending cannabis and other holistic healing modalities.

She is a psychotherapist, certified in psychedelic-assisted psychotherapy, educator, co-host for women's retreats, and entrepreneur in the cannabis industry.

Michelle believes in promoting caregivers' physical, mental, and spiritual healing. She dedicates this chapter to her dear husband, John Houston Bahel (09/20/1942-03/20/2024). She is forever grateful for his love for her and her sons, Lantz and Brandon. She is also grateful for all of their friends and family who unconditionally supported their marriage after the stroke. And she is grateful to Ethel Ried for being his caregiver and weathering it all with us.

Connect with Michelle:
Website: www.codegreenhealthcare.com
Facebook: www.facebook.com/Codegreenhealthcare
Instagram: www.instagram.com/code_green_healthcare
Linked In: www.linkedin.com/in/michelle-briggs-9ab549155
Email: michellebriggs@codegreenhealth.com

CHAPTER 19

Fill Your Life with New Experiences

HOW TO GO ON VACATION WITH YOUR LOVED ONE

Dr. Carol Sargent

MY STORY

Jim entered the calm and peaceful Victorian vacation home, grasping his bright blue cool box tightly in his right hand, with a weary look on his face. I was relieved to see him. I wasn't sure he would actually arrive.

Sylvia bounced up the steps just behind him with her bright red Tartan Hat and a beaming red-lipped smile.

She immediately rushed up to me,

"Hello, I'm Sylvia, I'm such a lucky lady to be married to my Mr. Wallace."

Then she turned and gave Jim a big affectionate hug, which showed us all just how much she loved him.

Jim tensed and looked embarrassed about her very public show of affection. I quickly started chatting to Sylvia.

"You're a very lucky lady to have found your Mr. Wallace. Was your lovely red tartan hat a present from Mr. Wallace?"

"It was. Do you know it's Wallace Tartan? I love it. I have a Wallace Tartan rug and cushions at home to remind me of my super duper husband."

I told Sylvia my favorite Scottish dance was the Dashing White Sergeant, like my surname, and we all started laughing. Jim began to visibly relax as he saw Sylvia and my colleague Amanda starting to hum some Scottish tunes.

Amidst the humming, Amanda said

"Do you want to listen to some Scottish Music with me, Sylvia?"

"Yes, Super duper," Sylvia said and followed Amanda eagerly into the dining room.

"Amanda, do you know I do 15 minutes of exercise each morning to my favorite Scottish Music?"

Sylvia promptly put her hand into her pastel tartan handbag and pulled out a handful of Scottish music CDs.

Out of the corner of my eye, I could see Jim starting to smile, and a look of pure, unadulterated love crossed his face. Sylvia was instantly aware of this and turned around and gave him her big, wonderful smile. Jim then let out a short sigh, and his body visibly relaxed.

He turned, and I saw his eyes had a sad, wistful longing.

"Gosh Carol, what a lovely place and what wonderful people. I would love to stay, but I need to tell you now, we'll be leaving tomorrow morning as Sylvia never settles anywhere new."

Then he finally released his hold of the blue cooler box, and the floodgates opened.

"I'm so sorry. I should have told you on the phone, but I didn't want to put you to any more trouble. You're already cooking Sylvia different meals."

"Sylvia is very conscious of her figure and is even more picky about her food than I told you."

He tentatively opened the blue cooler box. Inside was half a loaf of white bread, an unopened pack of ham, tomatoes, diet coke, a bountiful supply of chocolate Maltesers, and a small bottle of vodka.

"We never ever go out to cafes or restaurants. We just can't. Sylvia gets upset if she doesn't get particular foods, especially if they're not served in a certain way."

"No problem," I said.

"You know my mum has dementia?" I said.

"Yes, you told me on the phone."

"Well, she will only drink sparkly fruit-flavored water when we go out. If she doesn't get it, she just walks out."

"Really, I thought it was only me who had these problems."

"Now, when we go anywhere, just as we are sitting down, I tell Mum I'm desperate for a drink, grab the menu, go straight to the waitress, and ask her to make a lemonade with a dash of blackcurrant and something for myself. Then I sit down and tell Mum they have her favorite drink, and we start looking at the food on the menu."

I explain how it's taken me a while to come up with this approach and how I persevered because Mum loves cake and I'm not very good at baking."

Suddenly, there is a look of realization on Jim's face.

"I would never have thought of something like that." Then he stares like I'm someone incredible.

Which slowly changes into a knowing look: you really do understand what I'm going through, and I think I'm going to trust you.

Then he begins to open up fully about everything he does so Sylvia feels relaxed and enjoys herself. All because he loves her beyond words.

I listen attentively and don't interrupt. I consciously don't look surprised at anything he tells me, particularly as I asked many of these questions when we chatted on the phone, and he said nothing.

He explained everything except the vodka in the cooler box.

"I'm curious, is the vodka in the cool box something for Sylvia, too?

"No, no," he says.

"Sylvia goes to bed very early, and when I know she is asleep, I pour myself a vodka and coke before sitting down to watch TV. A wee vodka makes it easier for me to relax."

"Okey dokey, shall I put the ham and tomatoes in the fridge to keep them cool?"

"Oh no," he says. "You'll only have to get them tomorrow when we leave, no point giving you extra work. It's an electric cool box and I just plug it in the bedroom. You know it used to stop me getting to sleep, but now it's a comforting sound in a new room."

As we're stood chatting, Sylvia and Amanda scoot past us in the hall, smiling and laughing to join everybody in the living room.

Jim and I pop our heads around the door. Much to his surprise, he sees Sylvia relaxed, sitting on the pale yellow sofa next to Amanda, chatting away to everybody in the room.

"I just love Scottish music. My favorite tune is My Bonnie Lies Over the Ocean, but I changed the words to 'My Jimmy Lies Over the Ocean.'"

At that point, Jim interrupts her.

"Super to meet you all. I see you have already met my lovely wife, Sylvia. I'm her Mr. Wallace, and we are really looking forward to getting to know you all. However, I'm really not sure we will manage to stay the full week."

Sylvia looks bemused.

"Oh Jim, I hope we can stay. It's such a lovely place, and everything is ace. Amanda did Highland dancing competitions and is joining me with my exercises tomorrow morning."

The other carers give Jim a knowing look, and I realize they are all just as nervous as Jim and worried that they, too, may have to leave.

Then, all at once, the atmosphere in the room changes; the carers are sitting more comfortably, and they look more reassured.

I realize everyone is equally anxious—worried they might have to go home early and uncertain about what to expect in this beautiful, strange new place with people they have never met before.

As I leave the living room, I hear them all chatting away in a much friendlier way, eager to get to know one another, as they all now have that common bond: dementia.

I check all the shopping so I'm confident I can cook tonight's dinner and tomorrow's breakfast and then I pause to reflect on Jim and Sylvia's arrival.

"I'm just popping down the road as I forgot to order the vinegar to make tonight's Raspberry Pavlova. Would anybody like me to put an order in for newspapers for the morning?"

Pat chips in, "Frank likes his Sudoku in the Telegraph every morning. I've brought our vouchers." Frank gives her hand a squeeze and throws me a smile to say thanks.

Isabel pipes up, "Bill always has a packet of fudge at home."

She turns toward Bill, who's been sitting quietly in his chair, taking everything in.

"Would you like Carol to get you some fudge?"

In his deep, calm voice, Bill answers, "Yes, please, just plain fudge, no chocolate. The Original Fudge Company is my favorite."

Sylvia then joins in, "I'd love a packet of Maltesers. Do you know, because they have air in the middle, they don't make you fat?"

Everybody laughs, as this was the advertising slogan used on the TV.

Sylvia, nestles into her seat, comfortable she is now in a room full of friends.

Off I went, not to get any vinegar. That was a white lie! I was going to get tomatoes to go with Sylvia's Chicken Nuggets, plus some Diet Coke and Maltesers for her pudding.

A very embarrassed Jim also told me, "I'm so sorry, Sylvia won't eat any puddings, including my favorite, raspberry pavlova. She worries about her figure."

After a successful shopping trip, I get on with cooking dinner. Twenty minutes before the cottage pie was ready, I popped Sylvia's four chicken nuggets and two potato croquets into the oven, just as Jim told me on the phone.

When everybody entered the dining room, there were gasps as everybody admired the homemade place cards and beautiful napkins Amanda folded with Sylvia's help. Frank had a lovely glass of red wine waiting for him, which he was very pleased about, and Bill sat down and immediately took a long, slow drink of his beer. Sylvia was thrilled when she found her name card, a glass of Diet Coke, and Amanda sitting next to her.

I plated Sylvia's meal first, with her tomato quartered, just how she liked it. On a separate plate, I had a special surprise: two potato smiley faces.

Amanda served Sylvia her chicken nuggets, tomatoes, and potato croquets.

"Super duper," Sylvia said as she eagerly popped a quartered tomato onto her fork.

Just behind, I came through with the steaming cottage pie topped with golden crusty cheese to a loud chorus of "That smells delicious."

While all eyes were on the steaming hot pie, Amanda whispered in Sylvia's ear to see if she would like to try something special.

Immediately, we all heard Sylvia say, "Yes, please."

Amanda entered the kitchen and returned with the potato smiley faces on the side plate. Sylvia's grin stretched from ear to ear. Somebody had given her something extra special.

Amanda and Sylvia sat and chatted, giggling about the exercises they were planning for the morning. Jim was speaking to Pat about why she had moved to Scotland, and so our first dinner together started.

In just a short time, we'd learned it wasn't just dementia that connected us. It was more than that; we'd gained trust and confidence in one another, and we were collectively willing each other to stay till the end of the vacation.

I looked around and realized we were already one big, happy, dysfunctional family!

Much to Jim's surprise, Sylvia had a thin slither of my raspberry Pavlova.

He gasped as she scraped her plate clean and asked for some more. His smile lit up the whole room.

Everybody except Jim, Sylvia, and Amanda were going to the music concert at the local theatre after dinner. Jim had made their excuses, saying, "We need an early night. We've had such a long and tiring journey."

However, I knew this wasn't exactly true. It was so Sylvia could have an early night, and he could get her settled in her new bedroom, giving them the best possible chance of staying longer on the vacation he desperately wanted to have.

As we were getting ready to go out the door to the concert, Amanda, Jim, and Sylvia were snuggled on the settee, with Sylvia resting her head gently on Jim's chest while they watched her favorite TV program.

I marched into the living room with a tray held high, hiding my other special purchase. On it was a small vodka and Coke for Jim and the uneaten bowl of Maltesers for Sylvia.

"Thought you might like these while watching TV."

"You shouldn't have done that," said Jim.

"Don't be daft; we want this to feel like a home from home where you can both be spoilt."

"I know he said with a sad smile on his face. I really hope we're able to stay for the rest of the week."

This holiday marked the first of Jim and Sylvia's nine vacations with us over four years. Halfway through the vacation all three couples asked if they could go away together at Christmas. In November that year, we met up for a Christmas vacation in Yorkshire, and everybody had a "super duper time."

Sadly, Sylvia has now passed away. I was honored to give a eulogy at her funeral. It was a beautiful clear blue day, and the whole congregation sang her favorite song to her beloved Mr. Wallace, "My Jimmy lies over the ocean."

I keep in touch with Jim regularly, wishing him a happy birthday and seeing how he's doing. He's been an incredible advocate for people living with dementia and their family carers, sharing his experience and encouraging others to take the risk and go on vacation.

I share Jim's view. I want people living with dementia, their families, and friends to have more confidence to take the vacation they're longing for.

I want people in the dementia community and others with similar barriers to experience the freedom and joy of meeting new people, trying new experiences, and spending quality time with the people they love through travel.

When I'm speaking with someone who is considering a vacation, the first step is to understand why a vacation is important and what a successful vacation would look like to them.

By asking the right questions, listening attentively, and showing no judgment, we build trust, and a relationship begins to grow. This allows us to move on to the next step: identifying the barriers to going on vacation.

We capture everything together before separating the information into what's within our control, what's not, and where we might be able to provide support to lessen those barriers.

We explore the things we can't control and discuss what we could do if this actually happened on vacation. We work together to decide on an approach to managing the situation and come up with realistic solutions, reassuring everybody that everything is being thought of.

When identifying a concern, I often ask my clients, "Are you willing to take the risk and manage this situation on the vacation you're wanting to go on?" If the answer is yes, we capture the concern along with the solution and continue on.

If the answer is no, I ask my client, "Can you think of another type of vacation where you could manage this situation?"

If the answer is yes, I ask them both, "Do you want to go on this kind of vacation?" If the answer is no, then we mutually agree they are not ready to go on vacation at the moment. We then reflect on our discussion and consider other options.

As we go through this process, we paint a picture together of the vacation they are confident to take. We also capture a list of the things that need to be in place to enable them to comfortably spend time away from home.

At the end of the process, we provide our recommendations on the type of vacation and the most appropriate transportation and, most importantly, identify what support is needed to make their vacation relaxing. This support comes in different forms, from information, equipment, technology, or people, collectively empowering them to have the freedom and joy we all know we get from a great vacation.

Through these discussions, I notice how carers continually disregard themselves, putting their loved ones first and second guessing if they're doing things right. This isn't helped as, all too often, people are given the wrong advice about what you should do to support your loved one with dementia.

Everybody is told that maintaining routine and staying in your own environment is key. This completely contradicts the vacation experience and discourages many carers from vacationing with their loved ones. They know they will be in a different environment where it's harder to control their daily routine.

We all experienced the pandemic, the fear of something dreadful happening, and the desperation to change our routines and constraints. People living with dementia face these fears every day, which, over time, can cause isolation and depression.

I believe we need to recognize it's good for people with dementia to go outside their normal environment and have new experiences. Like everybody else, there are some they'll enjoy, and others they'll dislike, but fear of a negative reaction shouldn't stop us from experiencing new things. It should make us take more time to savor the moments someone finds joy in. It gives us the opportunity to learn about one another and how we experience the world around us.

This is all part of living—experiencing the good, the bad, and the ugly.

Family carers don't choose their role; it happens gradually over time. On that first vacation in Scotland with our three couples, I realized every single person was taking a risk, a step into the unknown. However, through getting to know them before and during their vacation, I understood these people were passionate about understanding one another to live their best lives.

THE STRATEGY

So, in ending my chapter, I'd like you to focus on five points to confidently take the vacation you're longing for:

1. What do you want from a vacation?
2. Remember a risk you've taken that gave you joy.
3. Look for solutions to your worries.
4. Don't be afraid to ask for support.
5. Live your best lives.

Lastly, remember that life is full of risks, and if we don't take them, we won't learn, and we won't know if we are living our best lives.

We love giving dementia travel advice at Sargent Group Consulting because we know the difference travel makes in all our lives.

For us, life begins at the end of our comfort zone, and that's often just asking for support and advice from people with lived experience.

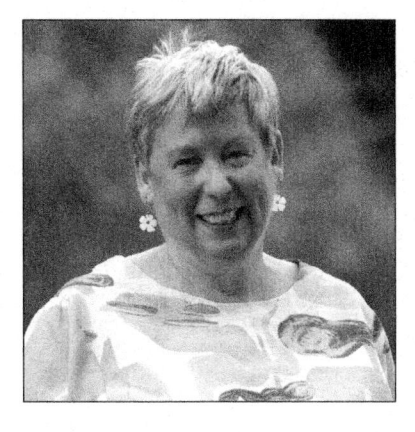

With her scientific background, business acumen, and hands-on experience with dementia, Carol has a unique insight into where dementia can intersect with travel and tourism.

Dr. Carol Sargent is Scottish. She lives in a village in Leicestershire in middle England with her husband, Gary, their cockapoo Darwin, and their black cat, Hugo. She has two grown-up children, Emma and Ben, who live and work in London.

She enjoyed a scientific career with international drug companies in the U.K. and the U.S. for over 25 years. Dementia joined her family in the mid-2000s and changed both her personal and professional life.

In 2014, she founded MindforYou, a specialist dementia vacation organization, amassing expertise in U.K. dementia holidays, contributing to the first Visit Britain Business Guide on Dementia Tourism, and generating the first independently validated well-being benefits from a vacation for carers of people living with dementia.

Carol navigated MindforYou through the pandemic and led its conversion to a charitable cooperative. In August 2022, she decided to step down as CEO and pursue opportunities to give the dementia community more vacation choices. In early 2023, Carol launched Sargent Group Consulting to support the dementia community in finding freedom and joy through meeting new people, having new experiences, and spending quality time with the people they love through travel.

In November 2023, she released her first book, Holidaying with Dementia: Your 10-Step Approach. An updated version has just been released and is offered free to members of her private Dementia Travel and Tourism Facebook group.

Carol continues to collaborate and work with various organizations to enable and empower the global dementia community to live its best lives while continuing to support her local dementia-inclusive community in Leicester, Leicestershire, and Rutland, England.

Lets connect at

Website: https://www.sargentgroup.consulting

Private Dementia Travel and Tourism Facebook Group:
https://www.facebook.com/groups/1364258777690947

Book Your Free 30 minute Dementia Travel Consultation:
https://sargentgroup.consulting/dementia-travel-advice/#enquiryForm

Download you free E-booklet:
Holidaying with Dementia Your 10-Step Approach
https://sargentgroup.consulting/dementia-travel-advice/#HolidayBooklet

LinkedIn: https://www.linkedin.com/in/carolsargent/

Facebook: https://www.facebook.com/allenby.carol/

Twitter: https://x.com/casargent1964

TickTock: https://www.tiktok.com/@carolsargent

Email: Carol@sargentgroup.consulting

CHAPTER 20

Massive Acceptance and Radical Presence

THE KEY TO POSITIVELY NAVIGATING YOUR CAREGIVING JOURNEY

Susan J. Ryan

"Massive acceptance and radical presence give me the gift of living each moment from its greatest potential."

~ Susan J. Ryan

MY STORY

As dusk began gently settling, the singing sounds of the birds wishing each other good evening interrupted the quiet of our lazy South Florida afternoon. My daddy and I sat comfortably on the patio with his springer spaniel, Cricket, sleeping peacefully between us.

Suddenly, Daddy jumped up, calling out, "Walk the dog."

Startled, Cricket leaped up and began jumping around. In what seemed like an instant, Daddy grabbed her leash off the table, fastened it to her collar, and headed toward one of the two screen doors that led out of the patio.

My parent's home was at the top of a sloping grassy hill covered in the rough and coarse St. Augustine grass native to where we live. The door Daddy was headed toward led onto this grass, ending at the bottom of the hill where a concrete walking path circled the neighborhood lake.

I went instantly from peacefully relaxed to full-out frightened. Like Cricket, I, too, leaped up startled! Daddy had already taken several steps before I could get my bearings.

LIFE LESSON ONE

So many times throughout my life, my daddy has taught me two types of lessons. Focusing on safety began with him saying, "I want to teach you how to be safe in case I'm not here to help you."

Now, it was my turn to keep him safe. I knew he was about to make an unsafe choice—walking down the uneven, grassy hill at dusk with a startled dog pulling at her leash as she bounded quickly back and forth. Seemingly all coming simultaneously, my mind conjured up many potential disasters that could result if Daddy and Cricket went this way.

The patio had a door on each side—the one daddy was headed out, and the one on the other side opened onto the concrete path from their home leading down to the walking path around the lake. I ran to Daddy, stood before him, pointed in the other direction, and said, "Daddy, Daddy, let's go this other way. It's safer."

He kept going.

Continuing to worry about all that could go wrong, I tried again. "Daddy, please, let's go this way. It's safer."

Then, the unimaginable happened.

My daddy, the kindest, gentlest man in my life, pushed me out of the way to go out the door!

For an instant, I froze in complete shock.

Quickly gathering myself, I caught up with him as he walked down the hill. I stayed close to Daddy and got close to Cricket's leash in case he stumbled on the rough grass or Cricket pulled him off balance. As we walked down the hill, my eyes darted back and forth like a hunter, surveying the grass for anything that could cause him harm.

We ultimately made it safely (though not calmly) onto the paved path. My daddy was agitated. The dog was agitated. I was agitated.

I knew there was a powerful lesson in this experience.

Later that evening, I sat quietly, reflecting on what had happened. I felt a mixture of disappointment, anger, and concern. I felt disappointed for not being there for him when he'd always been there for me, angry at what the disease was taking from him, and concerned about how unprepared I was to help him. I was emotionally exhausted from the experience. I knew I had let my Daddy down.

LIFE LESSON TWO

I then used the second type of lesson Daddy taught. This one began with, "I want to teach you how to think so you'll know what to do when I'm not here for you."

Growing up, as he said this to me repeatedly, it never occurred to me that I might be using this lesson on my own - while he was still alive.

My daddy was living with the diagnosis of a type of dementia. I accepted this. By the time of his diagnosis, I'd already been in a variety of family caregiving roles. It was while caring for my daddy, during this experience when I felt I was letting him down, that he taught me my most valuable life lesson.

I'd accepted my daddy had a type of dementia, and yet I hadn't *completely* accepted it. I was judging what he was doing through the lens of what he'd modeled for me, what he'd taught me all my life. I was present to what he was trying to do, yet I wasn't *fully* present. If I had been, I would've known he was already doing what he had access to.

In that moment of reflection, massive acceptance and radical presence revealed themselves to me.

THE STRATEGY

Massive acceptance is accepting exactly what is, 100 percent. We don't have to like it. We don't have to agree with it. We don't have to understand it in the moment. We just have to accept this *is* exactly what it is, without judgment of ourselves, the situation, or others.

Radical presence is staying fully present in *this* moment. We're not wishing it was the way it had been and we're not fortune-telling into the future.

Through massive acceptance and radical presence, I let go.

I let go of wanting the familiar past, where my daddy constantly taught me to be safe and how to think. I accepted fully and completely that he could no longer access these or make wise choices independently.

With massive acceptance and radical presence—and without judgment—I now journey as the observer, not the judge. I stay fully present in the moment, moment by moment. As the observer, I'm at choice about my thoughts, my feelings, and my actions.

You may have heard the expression 'History repeats itself.'

A few months after the experience with my daddy, my husband, Jack, was diagnosed with a type of dementia.

OUR JOURNEY IS DIFFERENT

Living through massive acceptance and radical presence, so very much is different with our journey, beginning with the diagnosis.

The diagnosis is what it is.

Jack and I were in the doctor's office, sitting quietly next to each other, holding hands with our fingers intertwined. We were at peace with whatever the doctor shared because we fully accepted what we'd learn.

When we heard the office door begin to open, we smiled at each other and gently squeezed each other's hands. As the doctor shared the diagnosis, Jack and I began a new path on our journey of love.

Jack consciously chose to accept this journey for as long as he could choose. When he no longer could choose, I chose for him.

THE PRESENT MOMENT

In his 2005 book, *Being Peace*, global spiritual leader, poet, and peace activist Thich Nhat Hanh wrote, "Breathing in, I calm body and mind. Breathing out, I smile. Dwelling in the present moment I know this is the only moment."

Being fully, radically present, I have access to the potential and possibilities in each moment, moment by moment. I'm able to make the wisest choices in the most challenging moments, I'm able to see beauty in the tiniest moments, and I'm able to stay at peace in each situation.

THE WISEST CHOICES

In August 2017, Hurricane Irma was forecast to come on shore as a category four storm where we lived in Naples, Florida. Every news outlet, weather reporter, and weather app prioritized information about potential significant damage. Jack's diagnosis had advanced to where I knew I could put us both at risk if we stayed.

I immediately evacuated. I called family in Atlanta, packed the car, made a reservation at a hotel partway there, and, within two hours, we began our journey. The house and its contents were "stuff." Our safety was the top priority. As I closed the front door, I said goodbye to them. I was at peace.

THE TINIEST MOMENTS

I feel joy in the simplest, the tiniest of moments.

As his diagnosis progressed, I moved Jack into a memory care unit. Musicians frequently visited, playing songs that stimulated residents' memories. Family members were also there, and we all enjoyed seeing how the music positively touched each person.

For one resident, Amanda, her disease had progressed to the point where she was no longer able to communicate. She had minimal ability to show expression or move her hands and feet.

One day, the musician who came in played quite energetic songs; most of us were singing and moving along with the music. I looked over and saw Amanda's foot tapping ever so slightly. Joyfully, I shared this with everyone in our group. We were all so excited you'd have thought we'd just won the lottery.

We chose to focus on the beauty of this tiny movement and have a positive experience rather than on what Amanda didn't have access to.

THE POWER OF CHOICE

I had two goals for every component of Jack's care; everything we did was through the lens of him being safe and happy. I shared these with each person who contributed to his care. Aligned with massive acceptance and radical presence, they simplified our conversations, choices, actions, and emotions.

I still experienced each emotion. One of the greatest gifts of living from massive acceptance and radical presence is feeling the emotion that matches the experience, not the emotion fueled by judgment.

For example, when I judged my experiences with my daddy, I wasn't able to see them for what they were. I learned my anger at the disease was actually grief. Once I learned this, I was able to process my grief and move forward.

Through massive acceptance and radical presence, I shifted from feeling frustrated, overwhelmed, and, yes, sometimes frightened to confident, balanced, and supported in my journey.

STAYING AT PEACE

When Jack's health took a decline, I reached out to our hospice nurse. We recognized it was time to move him into the hospice facility for his final days of rest before his birthday into heaven. He'd be at peace and not in pain. With massive acceptance and radical presence, I, too, was at peace and not in pain. With our fingers intertwined, I felt blessed to be holding hands as he took his final breath in this life.

CAREGIVING DOESN'T DISCRIMINATE

No one thing prepares us for this journey.

We plan so many things in our lives: school, finances, weddings, children, trips, careers. We don't plan for our journey as caregiver and care receivers.

Neither diagnoses nor caregiving discriminates. They don't pick and choose us based on our age, ethnicity, race, religion, financial position, politics, gender, occupation, or family.

Our journey doesn't come with a roadmap of exactly what to do and when, and no one can take our journey for us.

Christopher Reeve was an actor, director, author, activist, husband, and father. On May 27, 1995, Reeve was paralyzed from the shoulders down after being thrown from a horse during an equestrian competition. He passed away in 2004. Christopher's wife, Dana, was the mother to their son William. She was also an actress. Dana passed away from lung cancer in 2006. Christopher and Dana modeled the very best of massive acceptance and radical presence as they shared perspectives of their journey.

CHRISTOPHER:

"At first, dreams seem impossible, then improbable, and eventually inevitable. Don't give up. Don't lose hope. Don't sell out. Either you decide to stay in the shallow end of the pool, or you go out in the ocean. Some people are walking around with full use of their bodies and they're more paralyzed than I am."

DANA:

"Some of the choices in life will choose you. How you face those choices, these turns in the road, with what kind of attitude, more than the choices themselves, is what will define the context of your life. Be brave. Be open-minded. Be kind. Be forgiving. Be generous. Be optimistic. Be grateful for the many unexpected lessons you will learn. Find the joy inside the hardship. It's there. I assure you. And, too, be open to inspiration from unlikely sources."

POSITIVELY SUPPORTING OUR JOURNEY

Massive acceptance and radical presence support us in positively navigating our caregiving journey in many ways. They keep us from wasting time:

- With emotions that don't serve us
- With beliefs that aren't updated or aren't our own
- Asking ourselves, "Why me?"
- Feeling stuck
- Feeling frustrated
- Feeling overwhelmed
- Feeling frightened
- Suffering without support

Massive acceptance and radical presence support us in navigating the emotional roller coaster of caregiving. As we stay present and emotionally balanced, we learn to make choices that allow us to adjust quickly to sudden changes in our journey.

SELF-CARE IS SELF-LOVE

Massive acceptance and radical presence open us up to prioritizing self-care by recognizing that self-care is not selfish. It's self-love.

It's easy for us to shave off our own self-care as the responsibilities of our role increase. I learned this the hard way. I want you to learn faster and more easily than I did that no one can take care of us for us. If we don't prioritize our own care, we can become ill as well.

As the caretaking responsibilities of my daddy and Jack's care increased, I shaved off my own self-care to make more time for them. Here are two examples I'd tell myself:

1. I don't need to work out every day. I can cut back the number of days I exercise.
2. I can cut back a little on my sleep. I'll take care of (insert anything here) after they go to sleep.

While feeding Jack lunch one day, he dropped a potato chip on the floor. My lack of self-care had me exhausted mentally, physically, and emotionally. I'd lost most of what I call the grace of space—that instant between when something happens, and we intentionally choose how we think, feel, and act or unconsciously react, reply, or respond.

I say I lost *most* of my grace of space because, fortunately, I had enough left, so the words I shouted of my reaction to the dropped potato chip remained in my head—not on my tongue.

How could you be so careless? I've been working hard all day. I prepare your lunch, and you can't even eat it carefully.

This shocked me on so many levels. That's not how I would normally think (and *definitely* not speak!).

I gathered myself, gave Jack more potato chips, left the room, sat down shaking, and asked myself what just happened. Wow, this is what not practicing self-care looks like.

That day, I reached out for support to help figure out how to find time to include my self-care in my daily routine while maintaining Jack's level of care. The gift of that experience was so profound that if I'm ever tempted to shave off self-care, I remember it and take action.

ASK YOURSELF

These are several questions I ask myself regularly to support my being intentional in practicing massive acceptance and radical presence:

- How do I want to show up when I'm with my care receiver?
- How do I want to think, feel, and act when making choices for their care and mine?
- How do I want to feel as I navigate my caregiving journey along with the rest of my life?

- Can I make wise choices for my care receiver and myself when I feel frustrated, exhausted, fearful, angry, guilty, or sad?

FOUR KINDS OF PEOPLE

Former First Lady Rosalyn Carter created a powerful saying about caregivers.

"There are only four kinds of people in the world - those who have been caregivers, those who are currently caregivers, those who will be caregivers, and those who will need a caregiver."

Living from massive acceptance and radical presence, when you're any of the four kinds of people, you'll know:

- You're not alone on your journey.
- You're empowered to navigate your journey with your loved one.
- You have access to the answers and possibilities for your journey and that of your loved one.

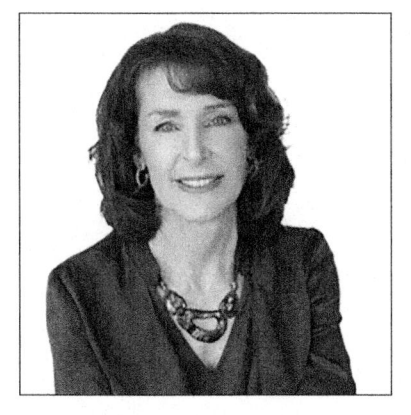

Susan J. (Sue) Ryan founded Sue Ryan Solutions and The Caregiver's Journey, to help you become your greatest leading yourself and others. She lives her life with joy and unquenchable curiosity about what else is possible. She has lived dual roles of business professional and family caregiver for forty years. As a speaker, change strategist, author, executive coach, podcaster, caregiving influencer, caregiving coach, and educator, she lives this through two passions of her purpose. She guides and inspires leaders and emerging leaders committed to business growth and next-level leadership to be great leaders of themselves and others. She guides non-professional caregivers to become confident, balanced, and supported in all phases of their caregiving journey. Sue is the world's luckiest Nana to five grandchildren and three great-grandchildren. She is a multi-time international best-selling author including *Our Journey of Love, 5 Steps to Navigate Your Caregiving Journey*, the creator of an award-winning online course, The Caregiver's Journey, a TEDx and DisruptHR speaker, and a volunteer for Avow Hospice. Sue and Nancy Treaster launched their podcast, The Caregiver's Journey and their book, The Caregiver's Journey, will be available soon.

Let's connect:
Email: sue@sueryan.solutions
Website: https://sueryan.solutions/
LinkedIn: https://www.linkedin.com/in/suearmstrongryan/
Facebook: https://www.facebook.com/TheCaregiversJourneys
The Caregiver's Journey course:
https://www.wcnuniversity.com/courses/the-caregivers-journey
Our Journey of Love book:
https://tinyurl.com/NavigateCaregivingBook

CHAPTER 21

Hospice and the End of Life Doula

WHEN HOSPICE ISN'T ENOUGH

Veronica Scheers, RN, CEOLD

MY STORY

An end-of-life doula improved the outcome of this story with time for bedside relief coverage, time for family gatherings to share concerns, compassionate listening, and time to review mortuary plans and memorial services.

FRIDAY, JULY 22, 2022 10:00 AM

The phone rang while I was on vacation. It was a stellar day on the Oregon coast, and I happily played with my energetic grandson.

You have a business to run. Answer the phone.

"Hello, this is Veronica," I said with a lilt in my voice. "Hello, I'm Karen, and I'm looking for an end-of-life doula. I'm reading a book called *The Book of Two Ways* about an end-of-life doula, and I think I need your help with my mom, Diane. I found your information on the Doulagivers Directory, and you're near me. My mom has terminal breast cancer and is in hospice. I'm working from home and taking care of her." You could hear the overwhelm and anxiety through the airways as she talked to me. "I'm away from the house with my grandson. Can I call you on Monday?" I queried. "Sure, thank you," Karen said with a lighter exhale.

SATURDAY, JULY 23, 2022 10:00 PM

If Karen is working from home there is no way she is available on Monday. Send her a text in the morning.

SUNDAY, JULY 24, 2022, 8:21 AM

Veronica: Good morning, Karen it's Veronica Scheers, RN, with Guiding Your Light at End of Life. The certified end-of-life doula you spoke with on Friday. I know we spoke about connecting on Monday; however, I wanted to text and let you know I am available anytime today if you are. With you juggling work and your mom, I thought today might be more convenient. Thank you for contacting me and looking for a doula for assistance in this experience.

Karen: Thank you for the follow-up. I'm looking for someone who can visit Mom in person here in Martinez. Do you only provide services remotely via telephone?

Veronica: Yes, right now, I'm living on the road in my RV. I use my Zoom channel to work with my clients. My home base is in Pleasant Hill, and I'm coming home next week for an unknown amount of time. I would be honored to help with your mom and stay local to be able to do in-person work. How about an introductory Zoom meeting in an hour?

Karen: I can try and pull myself together in an hour. Long days and nights with my mom, so moving slowly this morning. My mom is sleeping now, so I'll hop in the shower and get dressed. My email for the Zoom link is xxx@email.com.

Veronica: No rush. The room is open when you're ready, so please take your time.

This is how we started; we're on our first Zoom call. I'm in my RV on Cape Arego Highway in Oregon, overlooking the majestic blues of the

Pacific Ocean, smelling the salty air and hearing the waves crashing the shore while seagulls are flying nearby. Karen is in Martinez, California, in her home office just two doors away from her mother. The lights are dimmed, and she talks softly so as not to awaken her mom. She looks haggard and pale with bags under her eyes.

Over this free consultation, we discussed my 40 years of bedside nursing care, 30 years in critical care, my passion for my new line of work, and its importance in end-of-life care.

I informed her of what I would be providing:

- Collaboration with the hospice team
- Companionship to the dying and their loved ones
- Teaching any concepts given by hospice that the caregivers do not understand
- Suggesting interventions for comfort
- Help to facilitate unresolved issues
- Help with Advanced Directives
- Help planning the vigil
- End-of-life planning
- Writing the obituary
- Writing the eulogy
- Creating remembrances
- Finding peace and acceptance: helping the patient to find meaning in their life and what their contribution was to this life
- Support the patient and their loved ones through the entire end of life journey

I wouldn't be providing:

- A home health aide
- I wouldn't make any decisions related to end-of-life care for the patient directly
- I won't project my own beliefs and will always remain nonjudgmental

I listened carefully and compassionately as Karen explained how she had changed Hospice companies because Diane was not getting the care she needed. Diane hadn't been getting home health aide care for three weeks. An after-hours call was placed and no response was given. Karen identified that a lot of things were happening to Diane, and no one was taking the time to listen to her and support her through the process. They hadn't given her time to ask questions or to ask why something was happening the way it was.

We discussed Karen's support systems and Diane's lack of friends and attachment to family. We discussed Karen and Diane's religious and spiritual beliefs.

After our conversation was completed, the End of Life Doula Family Agreement and Disclaimer was sent to Karen's email. She agreed to an appointment the next Tuesday.

SUNDAY JULY 24, 2022 2:03 PM

Veronica: Karen, this is Veronica, and there is additional reason God put us on this path together. You mentioned you have a friend who is a chaplain with the VA. The End of Life community has identified that the dying experience for veterans is different than for civilians. Doulagivers has set up a 90-minute free class for caregivers of veterans. This class is coming July 27th. I would love the opportunity to share it with your friend. Would you mind sharing my name and telephone number with her, please?

Karen: Done!

Veronica: Thanks so much!

TUESDAY JULY 26, 2022 10:39 AM

Karen: My apologies for the butt call yesterday. I just signed the agreement.

Karen (2:53 pm): I'm available now if you are.

Veronica: I'm sorry, I'm in town taking care of some business. Would 5:00 pm work?

Karen: Yes. Do I use the same link from Sunday?

Veronica: Yes, please!

Our five o'clock meeting involved the changes Karen was seeing in Diane. Diane skipped a couple of meals since Sunday, saying she wasn't hungry. I gently explained how, as death approaches, the stomach begins to not want much food, and Diane's favorite foods could be offered in small, frequent servings throughout the day. Diane also started sleeping more during the day. A home health aide from hospice started coming and would continue to come two times a week for 30 minutes. A nursing assistant was hired so Karen could work from home and not have to worry about her mom while she was working. Diane became more and more withdrawn and was only speaking when spoken to. Karen looks a little more rested having the nursing assistant, and some of the Hospice frustration was resolving with the new company.

I can't wait. I need to get to the bedside now! Death is approaching sooner than Karen realizes.

TUESDAY, JULY 26, 2022, 8:01 PM

Karen: Hi Veronica. I usually turn the lights on in my mom's room so she knows it's daytime. I am with her now. Do I just leave the light off?

Veronica: It's your choice.

WEDNESDAY, JULY 27, 2022, 9:17 PM

Veronica: I have arrived in Concord. I'm available tomorrow afternoon if you would like some time.

Karen: Absolutely!

Veronica: Does 1:00 pm work for you? Can you send me your address, please?

Karen: Yes!

Veronica: See you then!

THURSDAY, JULY 28, 2022, 12:56 PM

I walk along the suburban street of Karen's home, absorbing my surroundings. The sun is shining with not a cloud in the sky. Birds are chirping. I can hear the cars from up the road. This is my time for grounding, leaving the outside world with everything going on to approach Karen and Diane's home in a place of service, compassion, and support. It's important for me to be actively listening without forming thoughts before they've finished speaking and to have no judgments.

I knock on the door and am greeted by Karen. She is casually dressed to be able to work and take care of Diane. She's having a hard time sleeping because she has been at her mom's bedside trying to sleep. She wants to be there for anything her mother may need during the night. "I don't want her to be alone," Karen says.

We sit together in an organized, comfortable living room with light streaming through the windows. Family photos and travel mementos scatter the walls. We learn more about each other and Diane's condition, how the family is interacting with Diane, their comfort level with her and their ability to stay at her bedside. I point out that if there is anyone who needs to come to visit, this weekend, it would be best while Diane is still responsive. Karen runs through the list of who needs to come.

I'm ushered through the hallway to meet Diane for the first time. Diane is lying in a hospital bed facing toward a partially shuttered window. Her face is pale, her eyes closed, her lips chapped and slightly parted. She's wearing one of her favorite lavender tee shirts cut up the back to easily get dressed with her favorite Eeyore blanket over her and her Eeyore stuffy toy close by. Eeyore mementos, pictures of Katy and Elizabeth, her granddaughters, and travel photos adorn the walls. Her favorite music is playing softly. Care-taking supplies are stuck in corners in a slight attempt not to be seen. A wheelchair and commode are stored in the shower (all items Diane is no longer able to use). Karen rouses Diane to introduce her to me. "Wake up, mom. Veronica's here to meet you." She acknowledges me with a nod. I get closer to her and tell her softly, "I will be helping you and your family as your transition approaches." She makes no comment and closes her eyes in dismissal of me.

We made arrangements, and a gathering with Karen, Terry (Karen's husband), Katy, and Elizabeth was held on Monday evening. The dying process and what to expect in the coming days were taught, and all questions were answered. A discussion of Diane's life and her impact on each of them was brought to life by the stories they told. There was laughter, and there were tears. We talked about the funeral arrangements, eulogy, and obituary, and all were in place. I took on contacting the cemetery for what could be included in Diane's coffin with her. A card was given to each of them if they needed any other support.

Diane spoke few words during my visits, one day stating, "It's taking so long," and the next day saying, "It's going so fast!" These were teachable moments for her.

I provided a time of holding space while the family went all together for a celebration of Katy's successful thesis application and pending graduation. An open time frame was given for this event.

Hospice wouldn't do this.

TUESDAY, AUGUST 2, 2022, 9:19 PM

Karen: My mom's feet are cold. She just spit up again. Brownish color with pieces of something.

Veronica: How is her breathing? Is she still taking ice chips?

Karen: She wanted to actually drink, then immediately vomited. Before that, her breathing was very light. I have to look at her chest to see if it's rising.

Veronica: Okay, she's still awake then?

Karen: Yes.

Veronica: You might want to give her some of the nausea medication from hospice. Then maybe recommend to her that since she is throwing up, it would be a good idea to keep her mouth moist with the sponge.

Karen: Okay, just did that. I gave her morphine an hour ago. No ice, just sponge?

Veronica: Just dip the sponge in ice water. Right now, I'd hold off with the ice. If it upsets her, tell her it's for her safety. You might want to call hospice about the changes. I don't think they need to come; just let them know.

WEDNESDAY, AUGUST 3, 2022, 10:00 AM

Karen: Why is she still hanging on? I can't take the roller coaster of this anymore!

Emotional support was given, and the family gathered at the bedside to be with Diane. The family stayed away while I stayed with Diane giving them a chance for a break from the bedside. Prayers and mantras were silently practiced at this time. Diane said she didn't want a lot of people around.

THURSDAY, AUGUST 4, 2022, 8:22 AM

Veronica: Good morning, Beautiful Soul! How is it going? I don't believe in coincidences; I do believe in miracles. I'm going to forward you an amazing email I received this morning from Suzanne B. O'Brien at Doulagivers International. There's a written transcript I feel Diane could benefit from. If it's too hard for you to read to her, I would be honored to do that. I am available at 1:00 pm or can become available earlier. Please let me know how I can be of service to you and your family.

Karen: She woke me up at 4:45 am this morning. She kept repeating things like "I don't want to get stuck," "Help me, Jesus," "I want to go," etc., over and over for almost two hours. I did everything I could do to release her, I told her to go. I called her by name as if I was God calling her home. She is begging God to end this life, yet here she still is, and she is uncomfortable too.

This would have been a good time for Karen to call hospice.

Veronica: I think the email I will forward will make a difference. Then I'll call you after my 9:00 appointment, it's only an hour.

THURSDAY, AUGUST 4, 2022, 11:21 AM

Veronica: Can you talk?

Karen: Now she's moaning, making noises.

Veronica: I'm on my way!

FRIDAY, AUGUST 5, 2022, 8:39 AM

Veronica: How is Diane this morning and how are you? Everything you asked about is allowed in the casket!

Karen: Wow, good to know! My mom is sleeping peacefully. She did mumble a few things around 8 pm last night, so maybe starting the clock over. I did ask her if she needed to forgive herself or anyone else and she said no. I'm holding on. Working since my mom is resting.

Veronica: Excellent!

FRIDAY AUGUST 5, 2022 4:37 PM

Veronica: Just checking in. What did hospice say today? Would you like some time tomorrow?

Karen: Nothing very different from yesterday, just to give her enough medicine to be comfortable. The aide will be here, which should hopefully give me time to rest and do chores.

SATURDAY, AUGUST 6, 2022, 10: 15 AM

Veronica: Checking in. Anything I can help with? Questions or concerns or anything weighing on you or the family that I can help carry? Much love!

Karen: Not that I can think of. My mom continues to sleep mostly peacefully, and I'm giving her morphine regularly. I feel calm right now. Thank you!

Veronica: Excellent!

SUNDAY AUGUST 7, 2022 11:05 AM

Karen: Hello, mom's breathing changed about 1:30 this morning. Less peaceful. Some clearing throat sounds; sometimes seems like she's struggling to breathe. Lots of noises as she's breathing. The hospice nurse is coming. I'll let you know what she says.

Veronica: I can come over if you want support.

SUNDAY, AUGUST 7, 2022, 2:12 PM

Karen: The nurse said she could go anytime. I feel in limbo again but I was able to lay down for a nap.

Veronica: Rest well. Call if you decide you need me.

MONDAY, AUGUST 8, 2022, 1:30 AM

"Mom just died," Karen said calmly through the phone but with a slight quiver in her voice. *Karen was well prepared for this.*

"I'll be there right away," I said, hoping there was a tone of reassurance in my voice.

"No, I'm okay. The hospice nurse is on her way," Karen replied.

MONDAY, AUGUST 8, 2022, 3:00 AM

Karen: Hospice nurse just left and waiting for mortuary.

Veronica: Sending love and light. Call me after you've gotten some sleep and we can set up a visit.

MONDAY, AUGUST 8, 2022, 4:17 PM

Karen: Just got back from the cemetery. It was a long process. Going to take a nap.

Veronica: Okay. Great job!

Karen had envisioned my role to be a support system for Diane, as she had read about. When the doula comes to the bedside earlier it could have been as she imagined. Coming to the bedside when I did, Karen and her family were now in need of support. Diane was involved in the progressive stages of death, and being with her without overstimulation was what was needed. Each situation will be different. Diane's hospice team did not notice Diane's feelings of loss of control and frustration early enough to help her. A doula will provide support and compassion at whatever stage they arrive to find.

THE STRATEGY

- When a life-limiting diagnosis is given by your healthcare provider, call an end-of-life doula sooner rather than later. Early interventions can increase the peace and quality of the dying process.

- When a hospice recommendation is given, act immediately. Comfort and support by the hospice team can actually increase your life expectancy by 29 days. When you feel that more time is needed for support or planning, call an end-of-life doula.

- When you're not getting a timely response from hospice, or you do not understand what they're talking about, call an end-of-life doula.

- When you're afraid to face the dying process of a loved one, attend a free Doulagivers Institute On Demand Level 1/End of Life Doula and Family Caregiver Training: https://my.demio.com/ref/498Bn68S6QtlKSTF. Then, call an end-of-life doula for support.

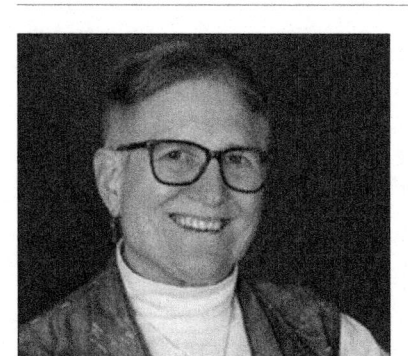

Veronica Scheers RN, Certified End of Life Doula, Founder of Guiding Your Light at End of Life, Hospice RN. She spent 37 years working in the same hospital with 30 of those years in critical care. On the cutting edge of the revolution of cardiac care and open-heart surgery. After 40 years in the art care of bedside care, her body insisted she retire. However, her head and heart were still a nurse. The good Lord placed in front of her an education opportunity as an end-of-life doula—everything hospice isn't. Since she had never worked in hospice, she signed onto a position her body could handle. The clients and their families appreciated her down-to-earth style and her meeting them where they were without judgment. She quickly saw what hospice wasn't and that management struggled with the amount of time she spent at the bedside. Because she gets such rave comments from the families, hospice can understand her style, and she continues working per diem while she builds her end-of-life doula practice.

In her free time, she enjoys traveling in her RV. She is 21 states short of seeing them all! She plays board games with her husband Peter, her Dutch souvenir. She is accomplished with adult coloring books, having colored her company logo. She stitches with her friends every week and has made 37 crewel Christmas stockings and counting!

Resources:

YouTube: End of Life University - Dr. Karen Wyatt

YouTube: Ask A Death Doula - Suzanne B. O'Brien

Barbara Karnes, RN - https://bkbooks.com

CLOSING

WHAT BOAT ARE YOU IN?

Debbie DeMoss Compton, CCC, CCA

What a powerful group of stories and information! If you're like me, you laughed, cried, and learned as you read. Each author shared from their heart in an effort to make your life less stressful, safer, and more manageable.

I hope you remember some of the main lessons. First, you are not alone. You may have heard it said we are all in this together, and while that's true, we aren't in the same boat.

Some may be in a sailboat, blowing from one diagnosis to another, one specialist to another, with tests and lab work thrown in between. You feel you have little control.

Some may be in a pontoon boat where the disease progresses slowly, and each day seems like a long journey. Day after day, you struggle with a routine you must maintain. You are tired and maybe depressed.

Others are in a speedboat with rapid changes and then times of balance followed by more quickly developing symptoms or behaviors requiring new strategies or solutions. You struggle to keep your balance, stay on top of new medications, and research new things to try.

Still others find themselves in a rowboat. You work hard but struggle to make progress alone. It's exhausting, depressing, and isolating. You long for help but aren't sure where to find it or how to ask for support.

A precious few are on a yacht with plenty of money and help to make the caregiving journey easier. You still struggle with the emotional pain of watching your loved one disappear before your eyes. No amount of money can reverse a terminal diagnosis. You long to talk to someone who understands your emotional journey.

And then there are the folks on a raft with no paddle. They don't know what to do or how to do it. Hopefully, none of you can relate to this one since you have read this book! If you still feel like it is you, email me, and I'll help you find direction. Deb@thePurpleVine.com

Please hear me when I say all these examples are typical. Thousands of others are in your situation. Hope and help are available, but sometimes you may need assistance finding it. That's where we come in. We have done our best to convey actionable information you can use.

Following this short chapter is a Resource Section. These are resources we have used and found to be reputable. They are national or global companies. There are podcasts, radio shows, an Elder Law Attorney, accountants, music and memory experts, consultants, doulas, teachers, trainers, and more.

I encourage you to scan the list and read the 10-word or less description to learn the main areas each resource covers. This is a goldmine of support! You can also scan the Q.R. code with your smartphone to access a digital copy of all the resources.

Apart from outside support, your mindset is essential in determining your happiness. If you feel positive and empowered, you'll have more energy, better focus, and clearer thoughts, which enable you to come up with creative solutions.

If you are depressed, defeated, and discouraged, it's nearly impossible to find workable solutions. By changing your focus, you can change your attitude and mindset.

"What are you talking about?"

Focus on what your loved one can still do instead of all they can no longer do.

"How can I do that?"

Mom had lost the ability to speak except for a random word or two that made no sense. I could easily be depressed, sad about all the conversations we could no longer have, or I could choose to be happy. I decided to find joy in this situation and still enjoy some moments with my sweet mom.

Kneeling in front of her wheelchair, I looked into her eyes and waited for her to see me. When she did, I puffed out my cheeks and crossed my eyes. She mimicked my actions, and we both laughed.

Out went my tongue as I tilted my head. Surprisingly, Mom copied my movements, and we had another good laugh. With joyful hearts, we hugged, happy to be connected even for a moment.

I am happy seeing her tap her hand and sometimes her foot to the beat of her favorite music. We used to sing it loudly and dance around like we'd lost all senses. Mom taught me not to care about who was watching or what they thought (something she learned when Dementia started taking over.)

It was hard for me at first. I was raised to act dignified, be polite, never call attention to myself, and be modest. Those attributes are impossible to maintain when you're loudly singing Johnny Cash's "Ring of Fire" and making wild gestures to accompany the music, dancing around with arms flying.

Seeing the joy on Mom's face and hearing her laugh again made all the embarrassment worthwhile.

Please, dear caregiver, for your sake and theirs, find joy in the abilities they still possess. Find joy in being together.

Making Mom smile became my goal. I no longer cared what anyone thought or how crazy I might look. It wasn't about them. It was about mom and helping her find some happiness in her day.

Strawberry shakes, ice cream cones, pudding, and chocolate made her happy. Who cares about calories anymore? Her time on earth was coming to an end, and we all knew it.

We did so many other things to make Dad, Mom, and my mother-in-law more comfortable, but I don't have space to go into them all here. You probably have some great ideas too, and I'd love to hear them.

Here are some statistics to help you understand my next point.

More than 53 million people in the U.S. alone provide care for an individual with some form of Dementia, according to the Alzheimer's Association.

- A meta-analysis reported that caregivers of people with Dementia were significantly more likely to experience depression and anxiety than non-caregivers. Dementia caregivers also indicate more depressive symptoms than non-dementia caregivers.
- Dementia caregivers report higher amounts of strain, mental and physical health problems, and caregiver burnout, according to a study of 1,500 family caregivers in The Gerontologist.
- Over half of dementia caregivers provide care for four years or more, significantly longer than family caregivers for people with other age-related diseases.
- People with Dementia typically require more supervision and are less likely to express gratitude for the help they receive (due to inability). As a result, caregivers are more likely to be depressed.
- Dementia caregiving increases mortality risks, even for healthy caregivers. Despite a significantly lower risk of mortality at the start of care, 18% of healthy spouse caregivers die before their partner with Dementia, according to data culled from the Kaiser Family Foundation's *Health and Retirement Study*.

Based on scientific data, the last thing I'll mention is critical, yet it's the one I still struggle with most.

Self-care is not selfish.

If you're like me, you may need to write that on an index card and post it on the bathroom mirror, the refrigerator, and the T.V.! Self-care felt selfish, so I didn't do it. I was a good little martyr for many years. My prayer is that you are smarter than me and that you take care of yourself and your loved ones.

If you don't care for yourself, how can you care for them? When you are exhausted, nervous, wound up, depressed, or happy, they feel it.

I've often seen a change in so-called "behavior problems" once the caregiver had a massage, soaked in a tub, went out for dinner, met with friends, spent time in nature, or did something they wanted to do.

When you feel robbed of the things you love doing, it shows up in your attitude and the way you care. Your loved one feels the resentment and reacts to it.

Do both of you a favor and take a little time for yourself. If you think that's impossible, respectfully, you're wrong. Here's an example of how I can make that statement.

I needed a few minutes of peace and quiet, some time I could decompress and unwind. I prayed God would provide a solution to my seemingly impossible request.

I was a family caregiver, alone with my mother-in-law all day. She didn't like the Daily Living Center and got upset at the mere mention of it. Other family members were at work or unavailable. *How can I fix this? There must be a solution.*

Suddenly, I realized that at my church, there are older adults who are cognitively aware and lonely. They would likely enjoy a chance to visit with someone.

After a brief phone conversation, I picked up an older lady I knew from church and brought her to my home to watch a movie with my mother-in-law. Their excitement was evident as they chatted and laughed together.

I gardened and relaxed in a hot bath to relax my tense muscles. It was amazing! *Why didn't I think of this sooner? It's genius!*

They were safe, enjoying an old movie, and I was nearby in case they needed me. Problem solved.

If you can't come up with solutions, it's okay. Don't beat yourself up. We all possess different talents, and problem-solving is mine. Your challenge is to reach out for help.

All 21 of us are here to assist you. We understand the journey as we've walked it, and most have gone on to get professional training to help you more.

You have our contact information, you know what we specialize in, and you know how we teach, train, and support based on our chapter. These authors have a wealth of information to share on a wide range of topics, not just the one they wrote about.

Please visit our websites, read our blog posts, and join our email lists if our style resonates with you. If not, no worries. There are more than 53 million caregivers just in the U.S. so there are more than enough for each of us to support.

If you prefer studying material independently and at your own pace, you'll love what I'm working on! I'm creating a self-directed learning platform. It has videos, written content, quizzes to solidify your learning, and a certificate issued after successfully completing the course. Prepare for more joyful days with effective stress-reducing strategies and quick anxiety relief. Enroll in my Caregiver Wellness, Stress-Reducing Strategies, and Techniques class now. https://thepurplevine.com/caregiver-wellness

We hope you keep this book and refer back to it as needed. It makes an excellent gift for a fellow caregiver too!

If you've enjoyed our efforts, please leave a review on Amazon. Reviews help instill confidence others need before they purchase.

Thank you so much!

We look forward to getting to know you and hearing your beautiful stories.

GO OVER,

GO UNDER,

GO AROUND,

OR GO THROUGH,

BUT NEVER,

NEVER GIVE UP!

~ Debbie DeMoss Compton

Resources

Resources listed are vetted professionals serving nationwide or globally. This list has been compiled for your personal use. It is not for duplication or for sale.

- **American Automobile Association AAA** / Offers senior driver course, insurance / https://exchange.aaa.com/safety/senior-driver-safety-mobility/
- **AARP** / Caregiver Resource Center / https://aarp.org/caregiving/
- **Aging Today** / Podcast focused on exploring options surrounding aging / https://agingtoday.us
- **Alegi Law LLC** / Estate Planning Attorneys / https://alegilaw.com
- **All Home Care Matters** / Podcast and YouTube show covering long-term care topics and issues / https://allhomecarematters.com
- **Alzheimer's Assoc.** / Helpline, online resources, support groups / https://Alz.org
- **Alzheimer's Speaks Radio** / Shifting Dementia Care from Crisis to Comfort around the world / https://alzheimersspeaks.com/
- **American Cancer Society** / Helpline, online resources / https://cancer.org
- **American Parkinson's Disease Assoc.** / Support groups, online resources / https://apdaparkinson.org
- **Angelic Sphere LLC** / Real time tech, for individuals, caregivers, families, & healthcare professionals / Angelicsphere1@gmail.com
- **Apollo Healthcare Company** / Take control of your brain health today! / https://www.apollohealthco.com/

- **Assisted Independence LLC** / Home and Community Based Services for Individuals with Developmental Disabilities / https://www.AssistedIndependence.care / limited service area
- **Assistex** / Games and Activities for Seniors with Dementia / https://Assistexstore.com
- **Assoc. for Frontal Temporal Degeneration** / Helpline, online resources, support groups / https://theaftd.org
- **Association of Mature American Citizens AMAC** / Offers defensive driving course, insurance discounts https://www.amac.us
- **Bridgetown Music Therapy** / Music programs serving people living with dementia and their caregivers / https://www.bridgetownmt.com
- **Caregiver Action Network** / Helpdesk, Caregiver toolbox / https://caregiveraction.org
- **Caregiver Chronicles** / Podcast for family caregivers / https://flow.page/caregiverchronicles
- **Caregiver Wellness Stress Reducing Program** / Online course to reduce stress quickly wherever you are / https://thepurplevine.com/caregiver-wellness
- **Caregiving Support Network** / Practical and faith-based support for caregivers / https://www.caregivingsupportnetwork.org
- **CareLink360™** / Simplest and safest way to keep elders connected and engaged / https://mycarelink360.com
- **Caring Place HUB** / Caregiver and employer apps, support, and education / https://carewisesolutions.org/
- **Chatting with Betsy Podcast & Radio** / Features topics and guests who offer resources to support caregivers https://passionateworldtalkradio.com/chatting-with-betsy_show/
- **Dementia Map** / A global resource directory to support dementia care / https://www.dementiamap.com
- **Department of Motor Vehicles** / Request a handicap placard / Check your state DMV to obtain a placard
- **Diane Marie Gallant, LLC** / Mental fitness and empowerment coaching supported by energy healing / https://dianemariegallant.com

- **DoulaGivers Institute** / Free Death Doula training to empower caregivers and families / https://doulagivers.com/
- **Echobox Memory Vault** / Capturing memories and elevating quality of life / https://echobox.ca
- **Eldercare locator** / Assistance in finding senior communities, caregiver corner / https://eldercare.acl.gov
- **Elder Care Solutions** / Empowering families with financial options to pay for care / https://www.eldercaresolutionsinc.com/
- **Family Caregiver Alliance** / Support groups, online resources, e-newsletter / https://caregiver.org
- **Family Legacy Financial Solutions** / retirement, estate, investment, and tax planning / https://www.familylegacync.com/michael-lewis
- **Guiding Your Light at End of Life** / Emotional, spiritual and physical support in collaboration with hospice / guidingyourlight99@gmail.com
- **Health Line** / The 7 Worst Foods for Your Brain / https://www.healthline.com/nutrition/worst-foods-for-your-brain
- **Lyft** / Provides individualized transportation, like a taxi / https://www.lyft.com
- **Mackenzie Meets Alzheimers** / Awareness videos for children and families; Picture book and song download / https://www.mackenziemeetsalzheimers.com
- **Memory Café** / Memory Café Directory, helpful tips for caregivers / https://memorycafedirectory.com
- **Memory Keepers** / Expert training, classes for dementia support / https://memorykeepers.org/caregiver-resources/
- **Memory Matters** / Memory assessments and memory improvement courses, global webinars for senior organizations / https://www.renayudkowsky.com
- **Mental Fitness Training** / Two free quizzes help you understand your mindset/ https://positiveintelligence.com

- **Mirador Magazine** / An award-winning, dementia-friendly publication / https://www.miradormagazine.com
- **Music with Alexis** / A dementia-friendly virtual music engagement program for groups and communities / https://www.bridgetownmt.com/musicwithalexis
- **National Aphasia Assoc.** / Aphasia is a communication disorder that impairs a person's ability to process language / https://aphasia.org
- **National Council on Aging** / https://www.ncoa.org
- **National Institute on Aging** / https://www.nia.nih.gov/
- **Neuroq** / KetoFLEX 12/3 Diet for brain health / https://neuroq.com/blog/what-is-the-bredesen-diet/
- **One Life Consulting** / Helping older adults navigate late life care challenges / https://www.onelifeconsulting.net
- **Parkinson's Foundation** / Education, resources, and support for people living with Parkinson's and their caregivers / https://parkinson.org
- **Patient Advocacy Foundation** / Financial aid, case management, Medicare resource / https://patientadvocate.org/
- **Primary Record** / Simplifying health information for better care / https://www.primaryrecord.com
- **Reiki Training** / Learn about the compassionate healing support of Reiki healing/ https://reiki.org
- **Reimagining Dementia** / A Creative Coalition for Justice; leading with creativity globally / https://www.reimaginingdementia.com
- **Relish** / Dementia-friendly activity products focused on bringing joy to life with dementia / https://relish-life.com/us
- **Resilient and Sustainable Caring** / Caregiver support and resilience, articles, newsletter, coaching, workshops/ https://karenschuder.com
- **Sargent Group Consulting** / Enabling and empowering freedom and joy through dementia travel / https://www.sargentgroup.consulting/dementia-travel-advice

- **ScrippsAVID** / Designed by the Scripps Gerontology Center to build social connections across the generations / https://scrippsoma.org/creative-caregiving-guide/
- **Singing at Home** / A dementia-friendly virtual music engagement program for individuals at home / https://www.bridgetownmt.com/singingathome
- **Sleep Foundation** / How Lack of Sleep Impacts Cognitive Performance and Focus / https://www.sleepfoundation.org/sleep-deprivation/lack-of-sleep-and-cognitive-impairment
- **Tea & Toast** | Senior living specialists, focused on educating families https://www.teaandtoast.ca
- **The 'D' Word UK Health Radio** / The UK's only weekly internet radio show about dementia / https://ukhealthradio.com/program/the-d-word/
- **The Purple Vine** / Dementia support, blog, weekly e-mail, free resources, books, consultations, training / https://www.thePurpleVine.com
- **Uber** / Provides individualized transportation / https://www.uber.com
- **Very Well Health** / 6 Ways That Exercise Helps Alzheimer's Disease / https://www.verywellhealth.com/exercise-benefits-for-alzheimers-98666
- **Whole Care Network** / Sharing authentic and diverse care stories with families everywhere. / https://thewholecarenetwork.com/
- **WillGather Podcast** / Navigating the World with Your Aging Loved One / https://www.willgatherpodcast.com/
- **Zinnia TV** / Videos that help people with dementia and their caregivers / https://www.zinniatv.com

To get this list delivered to your inbox, scan the QR code with your smart phone or go here to sign up: https://mailchi.mp/319bded1c697/resources

*Joy is always present,
sometimes we just have to look harder to find it.*

~ Debbie DeMoss Compton

Printed in Great Britain
by Amazon